Drugs
and Human
Behaviour

Gordon Claridge

Penguin Books

Penguin Books Ltd, Harmondsworth,
Middlesex, England
Penguin Books Inc., 7110 Ambassador Road,
Baltimore, Maryland 21207, U.S.A.
Penguin Books Australia Ltd, Ringwood,
Victoria, Australia

First published by Allen Lane The Penguin Press 1970
Published in Pelican Books 1972
Copyright © Gordon Claridge, 1970

Made and printed in Great Britain by
Hazell Watson & Viney Ltd, Aylesbury, Bucks
Set in Monotype Times

Contents

Preface

One of the satisfying things about writing a book is being able to sit back half-way through, or even after it is finished, to try and think of a title that will give the reader some idea of what the book is about. In doing so for this book I was aware that its title could easily have been 'Human Behaviour and Drugs'. For this is a book as much about behaviour as it is about drugs. Essentially it is an attempt to show how, by studying people given drugs, we can learn something about how drugs work as well as about how people work. I have confined the book mainly to human behaviour, for three reasons. Firstly, I do not feel myself competent to survey the field of drug research in animals. Secondly, even if I were, the inclusion of more than the few animal studies I have quoted would have made the book unwieldy and detracted from its main purpose. Thirdly, and perhaps most important of all, I decided from the very beginning that it ought to be possible to write a coherent story about drugs on the basis of what is known about their effects on human behaviour. The exception, of course, is the section I have included on drugs and the brain, where what little is known is derived largely from observations made on animals. The reader can quite happily skip that chapter if he finds it dull or too hard going.

During the preparation of the book several of my colleagues read individual chapters and I would like to thank them here for the helpful comments they made. I would also like to thank my wife for giving me a 'semi-laywoman's' view of the book, for help in proof-reading it, but most of all for her tolerance of my mood-swings while writing it. Thanks are also due to Miss Margaret Hagan for her very efficient typing of the manuscript and to Mr Louden Brown and his colleagues in the Department of Medical Photography, Southern General Hospital, Glasgow for their help in the preparation of the illustrations. Some of the diagrams are reproduced from elsewhere by courtesy of various authors and publishers. Their kind permission to do so is acknowledged individually on the page where each diagram appears. Kind permission to reproduce extracts from their publications was also given by Dr James Chapman and the Royal Medico-Psychological Association, Mr Jackson House and the Toronto *Daily Star*, and Logan Gourlay Publications Ltd.

Finally, a word about the drug terminology used in the book. Confusion often arises over the names of drugs because several different names may exist for the same drug. In order to standardize the terminology I have avoided the use of proprietary names and referred to each drug by its short chemical name. Since in some cases even the latter varies from country to country I have wherever possible used the name decided upon by international agreement. In this respect, I have been guided by the World Health publication 'International non-proprietary names for pharmaceutical preparations', Cumulative List No. 2, World Health Organization, Geneva, 1967. As a further guide to those

readers who are interested, at the end of the book I have included
a short glossary of drug names and types.

Department of Psychological Medicine,   GORDON S. CLARIDGE
University of Glasgow,
April 1969.

What is Psychopharmacology?

1

It is certain that some of you settling down to read this book are doing so under the influence of a drug. The drug may be one of the new tranquillizers that are supposed to relieve anxiety and help you concentrate. Or it may be a well-established sedative which also calms you but which, in addition, is intended to help you sleep (though not, I trust, before you have read a little further!). Both of these drugs will probably have been given to you by your doctor. Others may be self-prescribed. These may include that universal beverage alcohol or, if you are a student burning the midnight oil, the effective stimulant ingredient of coffee, namely caffeine.

What these drugs have in common is their ability to alter the individual's psychological state. They produce subjective changes in mood, thinking, and level of awareness as well as modifying the individual's observable behaviour. His responses to the environment may be sharpened, dulled, or, as anyone who has unwisely tried to drive home after a successful party will know, simply disrupted. Drugs that have effects of this kind – sometimes known as psychotropic drugs – form the subject matter of a rather recently developed branch of science called 'psychopharmacology'; or, as some with a liking for prefixes choose to call it, 'neuropsychopharmacology'. The latter term calls attention to the fact that the drugs in question are assumed to exert their influence on behaviour by acting on the central nervous system.

The fact that some drugs cause marked changes in behaviour has, of course, been known for centuries and the first experimental studies of the effects of drugs like alcohol were carried out many years ago. However, it is only during the last two decades or so that psychopharmacology has emerged as an independent scientific discipline. Its development has been very closely linked with advances in our understanding and treatment of mental illness and it is significant that the beginnings of modern psychopharmacology coincided roughly with the discovery of two drugs that are of special interest to psychiatry. The first of these, lysergic acid diethylamide, better known as LSD-25 or simply LSD, was found by accident in 1943 to have extraordinary effects on thinking, perception, and emotional response. The psychological state induced by the drug proved very akin to that found in schizophrenia. Although in recent years LSD has achieved an unfortunate notoriety because of its misuse by individuals taking it for 'kicks', serious study of the drug has helped scientists gain insight into the psychological changes found in severe mental illness.

Some years after the discovery of LSD's remarkable psychedelic qualities an important advance occurred in the treatment of mental disorder. In the early fifties the drug chlorpromazine, which had previously found application mainly in general medicine and surgery, was observed to have powerful tranquillizing properties. It was subsequently adopted as the first major drug that could satisfactorily control the symptoms of the acutely disturbed psychotic patient. The event provided a strangely appropriate complement to the earlier discovery of a drug which could produce psychotic symptoms in the normal individual. These developments in psychiatry naturally gave impetus to drug research. The demand for even better treatments led to the discovery of many new drugs having psychotropic properties, while advances occurred in the basic sciences necessary to the understanding of drug action. Thus, psychology, neurophysiology, and biochemistry all gradually developed techniques that made possible a more systematic study of the effects of drugs on the brain and on behaviour.

As psychopharmacology has expanded, so its boundaries have become more difficult to define. I said a moment ago that psychopharmacology had now become a discipline in its own right. It would be more true to say that it has become the meeting-ground for a number of disciplines having a common interest in psychotropic drugs. The diversity of its subject-matter can best be judged by considering the range of specialists who might attend an international conference on psychopharmacology. First of all, of course, there will be the pharmacologists themselves, at least those who have a special interest in psychotropic, as distinct from other classes of drug. As a group they will be mainly concerned with the chemistry of drugs, particularly their synthesis and mode of action. Then there will be a large, and rather mixed, group of scientists whose primary interest in psychotropic drugs is in using them as experimental tools for bringing under control and understanding a wide variety of biological phenomena. They might also be trained as pharmacologists, though the chances are that they will belong instead to one of the behavioural sciences, such as psychology, neurophysiology, or even zoology. Depending on the area of research in which they have specialized, their interest in drugs will range from behavioural to biochemical effects, observed in either animals or humans. A third type of delegate at drug conferences will be the clinical psychopharmacologist. He will most likely be a doctor, usually a psychiatrist, and therefore someone who uses drugs daily in the treatment of psychiatric illness. His contribution will include such topics as the therapeutic effectiveness of different psychotropic drugs and the problems associated with trials of new drugs in the hospital setting. Finally, some psychopharmacologists, again often psychiatrists, but sometimes social scientists by training, will be concerned, not so much with individual drug effects, as with the problems that psychotropic drugs have created for society, especially that of addiction.

Although all of these aspects of psychopharmacology will be touched upon in the pages that follow, much of this book is about drug research of the kind carried out by the second category of scientist just described. More particularly, one of its main aims will be to show how the study of drug effects can help the psychologist further his understanding of the psychological mechanisms underlying behaviour, in this case human behaviour. That being so, let us look a little more closely at the general principles behind behavioural drug research.

The rationale for using drugs to explore psychological processes can perhaps be best understood if we compare the procedure with another technique commonly used in behavioural research, namely the study of brain damage. There it is possible to investigate the function of parts of the nervous system by observing what happens to behaviour when these parts are removed or damaged. In psychopharmacology drugs serve a similar purpose, except that the lesions produced are chemical rather than neurological. Thus, behaviour is brought under control by administering a drug that is thought to have certain effects on the nervous system. By observing and measuring the changes that occur it may then be possible to infer what mechanisms are responsible for the particular piece of behaviour being studied.

Studying chemical rather than neurological lesions in research of this kind has some obvious advantages. An important one is that the lesions themselves are reversible and the effects they produce relatively transitory. This is especially valuable in human experimentation since it means that a wider range of behaviour can be studied than in investigations of brain damage. Since, for obvious reasons, damage to the human brain cannot be produced for purely experimental purposes, the psychologist has to rely on the study of damage that occurs naturally due to accident or disease, or as a result of surgical operation. In neither case do the patients studied represent a very typical cross-section of the general population. By contrast, the psychopharmacologist can investigate the behaviour of normal physically healthy people and, what is more, by varying the dose of drug administered, he can exercise a reasonable degree of control over its effects.

One difficulty that the psychopharmacologist does face, however, is that he may not know precisely where in the brain a particular drug is acting. He can sometimes only make a guess, therefore, at the nature of the chemical lesion he is producing. This is obviously rather less of a problem in animal work, where the effects of drugs on nervous activity can be directly recorded by means of electrodes implanted in the brain. Even so, the exact site of action of some of the newer drugs is still relatively unknown, and many animal experiments in psychopharmacology are more concerned with this special problem than with using drugs purely as research tools for studying behaviour. Here the experiments may have a slightly different emphasis, though studies of both kinds, those concerned with the changes produced by a drug and those more concerned with the site of action of the drug itself, are clearly complementary to each other and really represent, as it were, opposite sides of the same coin. In general the more knowledge that is gained about the site of action of a drug in the nervous system, the more confidently it can be used, in the way outlined above, as an experimental tool for investigating behaviour. For this reason more certainty attaches to the conclusions drawn from the results of experiments where well-established drugs are used. This is especially true of human investigations, since the effect of a particular drug on the human brain can usually only be inferred from evidence obtained using the same drug in animals. A typical experiment will help to illustrate how the psychopharmacologist proceeds to investigate human behaviour by bringing it under control with drugs and then drawing inferences about the mechanisms underlying the behaviour he has studied.

Supposing he were interested in the physiological basis of mental fatigue or boredom. One way in which he could investigate the problem would be to take two groups of people selected so that they were as similar as possible in most respects such as age, intelligence, social status, personality, willingness to co-operate and so on. Those in one group would be given a drug which the experimenter (but not the subjects) had good reason to believe would make them feel sleepy and quickly produce loss of interest in what they were doing. The subjects in the other group would be given what are called 'placebos', that is pills that looked identical to the real drug but which in fact contained a harmless inactive substance. This precaution would be essential because, as we shall see later, the subjects might react just to being given a pill to swallow. Forty minutes or so after taking their pills, all the subjects would be asked to do a simple but rather tedious task, like tapping with a stylus on a metal plate so that the number of taps per minute could be recorded. The performance of the two groups would then be compared and if his hypothesis were correct, the experimenter would expect to find that, in subjects who had had the real drug, performance began to deteriorate long before it did in subjects who had only had a dummy pill. He might reasonably conclude that the drug had a real effect on the psychological state of mental fatigue, especially if the subjects taking it reported feeling subjectively more tired. It might be possible to go a little further than this and draw some conclusions about the physiology of boredom. Supposing that work with animals had established with a fair degree of certainty that the drug used in the experiment had a dampening effect on parts of the brain that were known to be concerned with wakefulness, so that animals given the drug showed lowered levels of activity in that part of the brain as well as becoming behaviourally less alert. It might be inferred from this that these areas of the brain had something to do with what our human subjects experienced as mental fatigue and revealed objectively as a loss in the efficiency of their performance.

Of course the experimenter could have tackled the same problem in a quite different manner without using drugs, by manipulating the boredom level of his subjects in various other ways. He could, for instance, have tested the two groups of subjects at different times of the day, so that half the subjects performed the task when they were mentally fresh and the other half when it could be assumed they would be less alert, say in the evening after a big meal or better still after a long period without sleep. Another procedure would have been to have compared two groups of subjects who, although similar in other respects, were thought to differ intrinsically in their ability to withstand boredom on the rather monotonous task being used. For example, people who were rather extraverted might be expected to perform badly compared with more introverted individuals. Using drugs in this sort of experiment is therefore only one of a number of alternative procedures that could be adopted, although it is a particularly convenient method of bringing behaviour under precise control for experimental purposes.

It is possible, of course, that our experimenter drew entirely the wrong conclusions from his investigation of boredom and that the changes he observed had nothing to do with the drug's action on the brain. Supposing that the drug had some local effect on, say, muscles – so that tapping speed fell off because muscular fatigue set in rapidly. The subjective feelings reported may have been due to an experience of physical fatigue. These possibilities could be checked by carrying out another experiment using the same drug but a quite different task, one not involving muscular activity. The experimenter could also have included the additional refinement of measuring the subjects' brain waves on an electroencephalogram while they were performing the task. This would have given him an objective measure of the relative state of mental alertness in the real drug and dummy drug subjects. It would also have allowed him to discover whether changes in the brain correlated with the subjective experiences reported and the rate of performance observed during the experiment. Information of this sort would have helped to strengthen the experimenter's conclusion that the drug was having a genuine effect on mental fatigue.

In practice, of course, the situation is never as simple as this. For one thing drugs rarely have a single effect on the brain, but usually a complex action involving several neural circuits. Even where a drug's action is fairly well understood, its influence on behaviour will depend on many factors, especially the dose administered. Effects produced at a low dose may not appear at a high dose and vice versa. This dosage factor will, in turn, interact with numerous individual features of the organism. There may be variations in the drug response of different species, while even within the same species individual variability may be considerable. In the experiment described above the investigator would doubtless have observed that his subjects differed markedly in their response to the drug he had given them. He would probably have found that the tapping speed of some subjects actually improved, even though the average trend was for the drug to have an adverse effect on performance. These individual variations are themselves of considerable interest and later in the book particular attention will be paid to this aspect of psychopharmacology. In the meantime it is hoped that the reader will bear in mind that general statements made about drug effects do not necessarily apply under all conditions or in all individuals.

For much the same reason the classification of psychotropic drugs is at present somewhat arbitrary, since many of the substances studied in psychopharmacology cannot be assigned to rigid categories, in terms either of their site of action in the brain or their effects on behaviour. Nevertheless, as a rough guide, an empirical classification has been devised which groups together drugs having broadly similar properties. This classification will be described in a moment, but first let us look at the more general problem of how to define a psychotropic drug.

As we have seen, psychopharmacology is concerned with drugs that have psychological and behavioural effects. However, it is true to say that almost any substance introduced into the body can potentially influence the central nervous system and hence behaviour. Not all of these substances are of particular interest to the psychopharmacologist. Many drugs may produce psychological changes that are undesirable side-effects of their main action, which may be to deal with some physical condition. Those who have suffered the miseries of hay fever will be only too well aware that the treatment of this complaint can sometimes be as uncomfortable as the illness itself. This is because the anti-histamine drugs used to treat this and other allergies often produce drowsiness and lethargy as an unpleasant side-effect. Such drugs would not be considered psychotropic in the accepted sense, though it is interesting that chlorpromazine, a drug already mentioned in connection with the treatment of schizophrenia, first came to notice because of its anti-histaminic action. Thus it may occasionally happen that a drug used in surgery or general medicine finds application in psychiatry, and then passes over into the realm of psychopharmacology.

In general a drug can be said to be psychotropic if its main effects are on the nervous system and if these effects are considered of sufficient importance for them to be explored further either for purely scientific purposes or because they have real or potential therapeutic value in psychiatry. We say either scientific or therapeutic because, while most psychotropic drugs do find practical application in psychiatry, some may have little or no place in the treatment of mental disorder. This may be because more effective alternatives are available, as, for example, when a standard sedative preparation is prescribed in preference to alcohol. On the other hand it may be because no useful therapeutic application of a particular drug has been discovered. This is probably true of the hallucinogenic drug, LSD, which is of limited value in treatment. It is certainly true of strychnine, a substance that is of little use therapeutically but which, because of its powerful excitant action on the central nervous system, has been widely studied by experimental psychopharmacologists.

For practical purposes the psychotropic drugs can be classified into the six main groups shown in Table I, which also gives typical examples of each group, together with their principal effects on behaviour. Until the discovery of the modern drugs, classification was a relatively simple matter, in that a broad distinction could be made between the sedative/hypnotics, on the one hand, and the stimulants, on the other. Each of these two types was recognized to have roughly opposite effects; sedative drugs, such as the barbiturates, depressing the nervous system and causing drowsiness, and stimulant drugs, such as the amphetamines, exciting the nervous system, and speeding up mental processes.

Table I.   Classification of Psychotropic Drugs

Class	Main Behavioural and Psychological Effects	Examples
Sedative/ hypnotics	Lower mental alertness and bodily activity; induce sleep at high doses.	Alcohol Barbiturates, e.g. Phenobarbital
Stimulants	Decrease fatigue; increase mental and physical activity.	Amphetamines Caffeine
Major tranquillizers	Calm; reduce psychotic over-activity and excitement.	Chlorpromazine
Minor tranquillizers	Calm in anxiety and tension.	Meprobamate
Antidepressives	Stimulate; raise mood in mild or moderate depression.	Imipramine Monoamineoxidase inhibitors, e.g. Phenelzine
Psychotomimetics (Hallucinogens)	Cause profound distortions of mood, perception, and thought processes; simulate psychosis.	LSD-25 Mescaline

With the advent of newer drugs other categories, shown in Table I, were created. The tranquillizers are classed separately because, while they act something like ordinary sedatives, having a generally depressant effect on behaviour, they are supposed to do so without causing the mental confusion or clouding of consciousness associated with, say, barbiturates. As their name implies, the tranquillizers have a calming action and have been divided into two subgroups, the minor tranquillizers used to relieve neurotic tension and anxiety and the major tranquillizers which have a more powerful quieting effect in psychotic excitement.

The antidepressive drugs have usually been put into another separate group because it is claimed that they have the specific property of being able to lift depressive mood. Two distinct types of drug fall into this category. The monoamineoxidase inhibitors are so called because it has been suggested, although it is by no means certain, that they relieve depression by effecting a chain of biochemical reactions in the brain involving the blockage of the enzyme monoamineoxidase. A quite different sort of drug is imipramine, also classified as an antidepressive. The chemical structure of imipramine is very similar to that of chlorpromazine which, as we have seen, is classed not as an antidepressive, but as a tranquillizer and some workers have doubted whether there is really any difference in the action of these two closely related drugs. This illustrates how there are at the moment no hard and fast rules about the classification of the newer drugs, the present classificatory scheme being based on a rather untidy concoction of similarity in the effect, the chemical structure, and the therapeutic use of the various drugs.

In addition to the psychotropic drugs proper, psychopharmacologists are also interested in a number of other substances which are distinguished mainly by the fact that they occur naturally in the body and are not, therefore, drugs in the usual sense of the word. The best known of these substances is epinephrine or adrenaline, a hormone that is secreted by the adrenal glands but which can also be synthesized in the laboratory. Epinephrine belongs to a group of compounds called the catecholamines which, together with another substance, acetylcholine, are known to play important roles as chemical transmitters in the nervous system. They probably act, therefore, as chemical mediators of drug effects, since at the most fundamental level the psychotropic drugs almost certainly influence brain activity by altering the chemistry of nerve transmission. An example of this aspect of psychopharmacology has already been touched upon in discussing the monoamineoxidase inhibitor group of anti-depressive drugs. These drugs, it will be recalled, block monoamineoxidase, an enzyme thought to be concerned with the breakdown and regulation of epinephrine in the body.

As well as being important as chemical vehicles for the action of psychotropic drugs, hormones like epinephrine and acetylcholine are also of interest in their capacity to act as drugs. When injected, for example, they have a marked effect on blood pressure, heart rate, respiration and so on. They have sometimes been used, therefore, to study the emotional response of the individual, and when used in this way are joined by a number of synthetic drugs, such as atropine, which also produce bodily changes similar to those found in emotional disturbance.

Psychopharmacology is therefore concerned with a wide variety of chemical substances having an equally wide variety of psychological and physiological effects. In later chapters we shall see many examples of how the study of these effects can help the research worker understand more both about drugs and about behaviour. First, however, we must take a look at another fundamental problem facing psychopharmacologists, especially those working with human subjects. It concerns the so-called 'placebo effect', the tendency mentioned earlier for people taking part in drug studies to react as though they had had a drug even though in fact all they were given was a dummy pill or an injection of sterile water. This remarkable influence on behaviour of even the most innocuous substance is of considerable theoretical and practical importance in psychopharmacology and one which must always be taken account of in any consideration of human drug response. Paradoxically, therefore, the most appropriate point at which to start discussing drugs is with the question that will be examined in the next chapter.

When is a Drug not a Drug?   2

For most people drugs have some emotional significance and few of us can take them with complete indifference. If we swallow a pill for medicinal purposes we do so with the expectation that it will, for example, clear our headache or give us a better night's sleep. If we swallow it as a volunteer subject in a drug experiment then the fact that the experimenter has bothered to secure our services, and perhaps even paid us for them, will suggest to us that he, at least, expects our behaviour to alter. (And in this respect experimental subjects are remarkably willing to oblige, whatever you give them!)

Only part of any drug's effects will therefore be due to its direct action on body chemistry. The remainder will be attributable to factors that can, for the moment, be rather vaguely but usefully described as 'psychological'. The subject's (or patient's) attitude towards and knowledge of drugs, what he has been told about the particular drug he is taking, and the setting in which it is given will all contribute to the total drug effect. In this chapter I shall try to give some idea of the extent of this psychological component in drug response, to define the factors determining it rather more precisely, and to show how psycho-pharmacologists attempt to control for it in drug experiments.

Although all substances labelled as drugs are assumed to have some pharmacological action, in a significant proportion of cases – variously estimated at between twenty and forty per cent – the effects are probably trivial or incidental to the purpose for which they are given. Many doctors currently prescribing minor tran-quillizers, for example, are only too cynically aware that, in the small doses usually given, the beneficial effect, if any, of these drugs is probably mainly due to suggestion. In other words, they are acting as placebos, as substances medicinally irrelevant to the patient's condition and given to please or humour him.

This placebo effect was well known to many early physicians whose cures very often depended for their efficacy on the ritual with which they were dispensed. One eighteenth-century royal physician, Shaw, who himself seemed to rely more on psycho-logical than on physical remedies, commented [60]:

The principal Quality of a Physician, as well as of a Poet, (for Apollo is the God of Physic and Poetry) is that of fine lying, or flattering the Patient . . . And it is doubtless as well for the Patient to be cured by the working of his Imagination, or a Reliance upon the Promise of his Doctor, as by repeated Doses of Physic. The great Bartholine declares, he once, by Mistake, gave to a Patient a Bottle of Fair Water, instead of another Bottle of Liquor designed for an Emetic, and that the Patient's Imagination was so affected by the Expectation that the Water oper-ated as a Vomit.

The example quoted by Shaw is repeated many times over in the modern literature on drugs. Placebos given either as injections of sterile water or as pills made of starch or lactose have proved highly effective in the treatment of many illnesses. Apart from their more obvious ability to relieve mental symptoms like anxiety, placebos have been used successfully in severe asthma, persistent cough, diabetes, angina, seasickness, rheumatoid arthritis, and the common cold.

The potency of the placebo is seen even more dramatically in its side-effects, which can be as frequent and as unpleasant as in the case of pharmacologically active drugs. After taking a sugar-pill the individual may complain of drowsiness, staggering gait, blurred vision, urinary frequency, ringing in the ears, and a host of other symptoms, including, in one case, a severe itching rash which cleared up only when the 'treatment' was discontinued. As with active drugs, the frequency and severity of these effects will increase roughly in proportion with the dose given – though the lethal dosage of placebo is unknown.

Striking side-effects are not confined to patients receiving medical treatment, but may also appear in normal subjects given placebo pills in an apparently neutral setting. Some years ago I studied the effects of the tranquillizer meprobamate on the behaviour of a group of soldiers [12]. Only half the group in fact received the drug, the other half being given tablets that were identical in taste and appearance, but inactive. None of the subjects was told what type of drug was being studied and no hint given as to the subjective changes they might experience. A surprisingly high number of subjects taking the dummy tablets complained of unpleasant side-effects, usually of drowsiness and nausea. These effects were especially exaggerated in two of the soldiers, one of whom was so affected that he was unable to carry on with his normal duties and had to be withdrawn from the experiment and replaced by another volunteer. A second subject became so drowsy that he fell asleep on a park bench in a nearby town, missed a military parade, and was only saved from the guardhouse by my swift intervention on his behalf.

The results of this experiment also nicely demonstrate another feature of the placebo effect, namely that it is not confined to changes in the subjective experiences reported by the subject. It may also impair or enhance the ability to carry out objective psychological tests. The purpose of the experiment on soldiers was to see whether meprobamate had any effect on their speed of performance on a serial reaction time task. Here the subject was seated in front of a panel of five lights set in a row, each light being linked to one of five response keys. He was asked to press the appropriate key as quickly as possible whenever a light came on. This turned off the light and at the same time switched on another light to which a further response was made and so on. All the subjects did this task continuously for ten minutes and it was expected that the performance of those subjects who had received meprobamate would be slowed down relative to those who had only been given a placebo. In fact, there was scarcely any difference between the two groups, so we were unable to conclude that this particular tranquillizer had any real effect on performance. What was most striking, however, was that both 'treatment' groups performed well below the level of another comparable group of subjects who did the task under identical conditions, except that they had been given no pills at all (see Figure 2.1). In other words, just taking pills was sufficient to depress performance significantly. It is also interesting that the overall effect of the placebo was to slow down, rather than speed up, performance. Although none of the subjects was told what to expect, most of them clearly associated drug-taking with 'being drugged' or being made less efficient in some way.

In that experiment we were probably fortunate in picking a fairly simple speed test, because some studies have shown that not all psychological functions are equally affected by placebos. Some seem to be more resistant than others. In one Canadian study a large battery of tests was administered to a group of female volunteers before and after they had consumed placebo pills [43]. The tests included measures of visual after-effects, simple reaction time, speed at which the subject could cancel digits, and performance on a complicated track-tracing device. The greatest changes occurred on rather simple tests where speed was the main determinant of performance. Where accuracy was

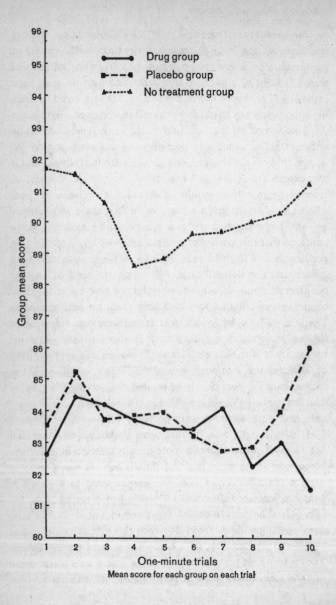

Mean score for each group on each trial

important, as on the track-tracer, much less change occurred. The experimenters concluded that simple mental processes are more sensitive to the effects of placebos than complex psychological functions over which the subject has some rational control.

In addition to their effects on psychological performance, placebos may also induce subtle physiological changes which parallel the subjective experiences described by the subject. For instance, measurable alterations in heart rate may accompany a complaint of palpitations, or changes in blood pressure a complaint of dizziness. Perhaps the most famous anecdotal example of this kind of physiological reaction to placebos is described by Drs Wolf and Wolff in an account of their extensive researches on Tom, a New York man whose stomach, because of an accident, was permanently exposed to view [74]. Wolf and Wolff had been interested in studying the effects of various drugs on the appearance and acid secretion of Tom's stomach. On one occasion they decided to substitute for the real drugs what they describe as 'three large imposing-looking red capsules' containing only starch and lactose. Shortly afterwards Tom complained of discomfort in his abdomen and the folds of his stomach became red and inflamed, just as they did when he was distressed. On another occasion an injection of distilled water caused a similar reaction, as well as a marked increase in acid secretion from Tom's stomach.

Even in normal individuals measurable changes in visceral activity can be produced by administering placebos with the appropriate instructions. In one study of this effect volunteer

Fig. 2.1. Illustration of a marked placebo effect on a serial reaction time task. Each point represents the average number of correct responses made per minute in three groups of subjects. The speed of both groups given pills, whether active or dummy, was much slower than that of subjects receiving no 'treatment' at all, indicating that just administering tablets was sufficient to depress performance on the task.

(Reproduced by permission of the publishers, *Journal of Mental Science*.)

subjects were tested on three occasions, each time being told a different story about how their stomachs would feel after taking a 'drug' [65]. On the first occasion – called the 'stimulant drug' condition – they were told that soon after taking the pill they would experience a strong churning sensation in the stomach. The second time they were given a so-called 'relaxant' drug which they were told would make their stomachs feel full and heavy. Finally, they were given a pill which they were informed would have no effect and which was being used as a placebo control to compare with the real drugs they had received previously. On each of the three occasions all that the subjects swallowed was a plastic capsule containing a small magnet which allowed the experimenter to record movements of the stomach. Out of six subjects tested four showed marked changes in stomach movement exactly in line with the instructions with which they had been prepared.

Similar placebo responses in other bodily systems, such as heart rate and blood pressure, can also be induced experimentally, as demonstrated recently by Dr Frankenhaeuser and her colleagues at the University of Stockholm [25]. Their study is particularly interesting because, in addition to physiological changes, the authors also investigated other features of the placebo response. These included an objective measure of reaction time as well as ratings of how the subjects felt after taking their pills. The subjects, all female, came to the laboratory on three occasions, the first time just to familiarize themselves with the experimental procedure. In one of the two following sessions each subject was given two white gelatine capsules which she was told contained a sleep-producing drug. In the other session she received two similar but pink capsules which were said to contain a stimulant. In fact, all of the capsules contained only talc. Measurements of heart rate, blood pressure, and reaction time were taken at regular intervals throughout each session and each girl was asked to say whether she felt subjectively quicker or slower and more or less alert, sleepy, happy, and depressed. The

results of Dr Frankenhaeuser's study are summarized in Figure
2.2. It can be seen that the two types of placebo had opposite
effects on all of the measures taken. Furthermore, all of the
changes were in the direction predicted. Thus, the 'depressant'
placebo made the subjects feel slower, more sleepy, and more
depressed, while the 'stimulant' placebo made them feel mentally
happier and more alert. These alterations in subjective state were
paralleled by changes on the objective measures. On the 'stimulant' the subjects responded more quickly on the reaction time
test and showed a rise in heart rate and blood pressure; while the
converse was true after taking the 'depressant' capsules.

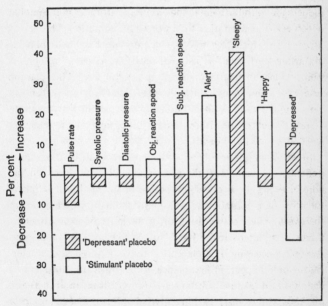

Fig. 2.2. Comparison of the effects of a 'depressant' and a 'stimulant'
placebo on various objective and subjective reactions. Each vertical bar
represents the average per cent increase or decrease in reaction following
administration of the two types of capsule.

(Reproduced by permission of M. Frankenhaeuser and the publishers,
Scandinavian Journal of Psychology.)

The two experiments just described, but more particularly the observations of Wolf and Wolff on the unfortunate Tom, are of value because they give us some clue about the underlying mechanisms of the placebo effect. Tom's stomach has been held up – metaphorically speaking – to thousands of medical students as an example of how emotional factors can influence the course of certain so-called psychosomatic illnesses – in this case gastric ulcer. Thus, prolonged anxiety, through its direct effect on bodily physiology, may aggravate an existing predisposition to illness. Placebos probably act in a similar way, except that when used in medical treatment they will work in the opposite direction, inducing favourable mental and emotional attitudes in the patient which will improve rather than worsen his condition. This is why illnesses in which psychological factors are known to play an important part, such as asthma, have on occasions responded well to placebo treatment. In more general terms, the placebo response – and many of the physical side-effects of placebos – can be understood as an emotional or psychosomatic reaction to certain aspects of the drug situation. Let us now look at the latter itself in a little more detail.

Most situations involving drugs are made up of three components: the drug itself, the person taking it, and the individual administering it, or on whose advice or instruction it is taken. Each of these components will contribute a varying amount to the overall effect of the drug; or, if the latter happens either by accident or intent to be inert, to the likelihood of a placebo response occurring. If a placebo is given, its physical characteristics would appear, at first glance, to be irrelevant, since it is by definition an inactive substance. However, drugs (and therefore placebos) can be dispensed in a myriad of forms that can scarcely fail to influence the consumer. They can come as hard white unattractive tablets or as pretty multi-coloured capsules. They may be administered out of large bottles as sickly syrups or vile liquids; or as injections which impress with their painfulness.

What psychological influence do these qualities have? Factual evidence is lacking on most of them, though there is some reason to believe that, under certain circumstances, placebos administered by injection may be more effective than those given orally. It is also believed that coloured capsules and tablets make better placebos than plain ones, though again there are few experimental studies to support the idea. Much of the evidence is anecdotal and based on clinical observation. This can nevertheless be quite convincing, as the following story, related by a psychiatrist colleague of the author, illustrates. For one of his neurotic patients, with a mild anxiety state, he had prescribed a common minor tranquilliser prepared in torpedo-shaped capsules, coloured half green and half black. At his next appointment a few weeks later the psychiatrist asked the patient if he thought the treatment was having any effect. The patient replied that he thought he was slightly improved, though he had noticed that he felt very much better on the occasions when he had swallowed his capsules green end first. The drug was clearly acting almost entirely as a placebo, though the psychological mechanisms involved can only be left to the imagination of the reader!

Given an impressive-looking tablet or capsule, an important influence on the placebo effect is the mystique and ceremony with which it is dispensed or, as Shaw put it rather more poetically, the 'fine Lying' indulged in by the doctor or experimenter. As shown in the experimental studies described a moment ago, quite precise physiological changes may be induced if the experimenter prepares his subjects with appropriate information about the kind of 'drug' being used and the sort of effect it will have. How effective these instructions will be may depend on other subtle factors in the situation, such as the relative professional status of drug-giver to drug-taker. Also important may be the surroundings in which the experiment is carried out, including any impressive procedures to which the person is subjected. In one study, for example, the subjects were asked to report any effects they noticed after taking what they were told was a harmless but pharmacologically active pill [24]. To reinforce the idea that they were earnestly studying the effects of a real drug and not a placebo, the experimenters wired a sham electrode on the subject's finger tip to a polygraphic recording device and pretended to be interested in the physiological effects of the pill. From time to time during the 'recording' the subject was asked if he had yet noticed any changes and after ten minutes, to increase the suggestion that the pill was genuine, he was told that the time of its maximum effect was approaching. As expected, the subjects reported a high incidence of physical symptoms such as stomach pain and itchy skin.

Often it is not necessary to go to such lengths of deception to obtain a placebo effect, though it has usually been assumed that one secret, at least, must be kept, namely that the drug is not really a drug at all. However, a recent study indicates that even this subterfuge may not be essential, as long as the appropriate verbal suggestions accompany the pill-giving ritual. The study in question was carried out by two psychiatrists at Johns Hopkins Medical School in the United States [49]. They treated a group of anxious outpatients with placebos in the form of pink capsules. The patients were informed that the pills were just sugar, that they contained no medicine and were quite inert; although some people, they were told, had been helped by this form of treatment. The patients were asked to take the capsules three times a day and to report back the following week. All fourteen patients who co-operated in the study improved, some quite dramatically. Over the whole group there was a forty-one per cent decrease in symptoms, as assessed by a symptom check list. This figure, the authors note, was actually higher than that found on previous occasions using a similar check list to test the effects of a number of proprietary tranquillizers. When asked whether they really believed that the pills were only sugar, eight patients said that they did; while the remaining six thought they had been deceived and that the capsules actually contained an active drug. The degree of improvement, however, was not related to what the patient believed but only to how strongly he believed it, whether true or false.

This experiment also draws attention to another problem in drug research, namely the *negative* placebo effect. It may sometimes happen that a person taking part in a drug study knows all about placebos and is well informed enough to realize that dummy pills are sometimes used for comparative purposes. In that case he may disbelieve what the experimenter tells him about the pills he is asked to take and respond to an active drug with the mistaken conviction that it is actually a placebo and therefore unlikely to have any effect. Alternatively, he may indulge in a guessing game, trying to work out which is the real drug and which is the dummy. An example of this kind of manoeuvre occurred in an experiment the author and a colleague conducted recently, comparing the effects of a placebo with those of dex-amphetamine. Almost all of the subjects were medical staff in our own department and were obviously quite aware of the effects of the active drug. The subjects had been informed what the drug was, though of course neither they nor the experimenters knew on any particular occasion whether the tablets were active or inert. (This was done by having a disinterested member of the staff administer the tablets.) Naturally, the subjects (and, it must be confessed, the experimenters) could not resist trying to work out what they had been given.* In fact, their guesses were scarcely better than chance. One subject, a psychiatrist of several years' standing, was quite certain after taking the placebo that he had been given dexamphetamine. During the next few hours he became more and more 'high' and the following morning announced that participation in the experiment had considerably enhanced his enjoyment of a party the previous evening. In contrast, other subjects were equally convinced that the ampheta-

* Since we were entirely interested in the physiological effects of the drug our own curiosity is unlikely to have biased the results, especially as we were invariably wrong!

mine pill was a placebo, dismissing as imaginary what were real physiological effects of the drug.

Negative placebo responses may reduce the therapeutic value of drugs, while guessing-game manoeuvres will certainly complicate the subjective assessment of their effects. From a scientific point of view, when measuring drug effects objectively they are not too unwelcome because a mixture of negative and positive placebo effects may help to cancel out the psychological component in drug response and make it easier to assess the real influence of the drug. Nevertheless, one hesitates to contemplate the double-think situations that may be created should any readers of this book agree to take part in a drug experiment or therapeutic drug trial!

If any did agree to become experimental subjects it would be safe to predict that some, despite their newly acquired sophistication about drugs, would show a significant placebo response to a dummy pill or capsule. Unfortunately, to decide beforehand *which* people would be placebo reactors would be a much more difficult task. Knowledge about the subject's previous reactions to drugs would not be of great help. Supposing, for example, they cooperated in a series of experiments carried out under a variety of conditions. The proportion of people showing a placebo response under the different conditions would probably remain a fairly constant fraction – about a third – of those taking part. However, this third would probably be made up of different people each time. Those who were placebo reactors in one experiment might not be in another experiment. Nor would background information about the subjects' age, intelligence, profession or social status help us very much. One would suspect that personality might be a better guide and this idea deserves a closer look.

What is the popular notion of someone who is gullible enough to be taken in by a sugar-pill and react to it as though given some potently active chemical? Probably that he (or more likely she!) is a weak-minded hysteric, an unstable character over-concerned with bodily health. The truth is that extensive research has failed to identify any particular 'placebo type' who will respond to placebos consistently under all conditions. Instead of looking for such a global personality type, recent studies have tended to concentrate on rather more limited aspects of personality, seeing how they relate to the placebo response in narrowly defined situations. Research of this type has provided some evidence that certain personality characteristics may be found more commonly in placebo reactors than in non-reactors.

One personality trait of obvious interest is suggestibility. It is almost self-evident that the placebo response is an example of heightened suggestibility, though it has not proved quite so easy to demonstrate experimentally that an independent measure of this trait is correlated with the tendency to react to placebos in the drug situation. One difficulty is that suggestibility itself is not a unitary characteristic, but, according to Eysenck, is made up of two unrelated components. One of these components has been named 'primary suggestibility' and refers to the tendency to react to suggestion with motor movements; as, for example, on the body sway test where the subject's degree of sway is measured under the suggestion that he is falling forward. The other component, named 'secondary suggestibility', refers to the inducement of feelings or perceptions in the subject. It is not entirely clear at present which aspect of suggestibility may be involved in the placebo response. One would expect it to be secondary suggestibility, though the few studies that have been done have mostly looked at primary suggestibility. When patients are used as subjects there seems to be some evidence that primary suggestibility is related to the placebo response, as the following study illustrates [64].

The experimenters set out to investigate how far the improvement of psychiatric outpatients, treated by placebo, could be predicted from their performance in the Press Test of suggestibility. In this test the subject sits with his eyes closed holding a rubber bulb. It is then suggested to him that his grip on the bulb is getting tighter and tighter. The increase in grip pressure under this suggestion is then a measure of his suggestibility. In the experiment concerned suggestibility was significantly correlated with a positive reaction to the placebo, the more suggestible patients showing a greater clinical improvement after one week on dummy pills.

Another somewhat similar trait that has recently been examined in placebo reactors is acquiescence or, as it is sometimes called, 'yea-saying'. This may be described as the tendency to respond in a way that is pleasing or acceptable to others. It occurs particularly as a response-bias in people completing personality and other inventories, in which the answer 'yes' may be given indiscriminately to questions, irrespective of their content. Thus, a personality scale of social extraversion might include a question such as 'Are you only at ease in the company of close friends?' The same question could be phrased in the opposite way, in the form 'Do you feel at home in the company of strangers?' The acquiescent individual may reply 'yes' to both forms of the question.

There is some evidence that in certain situations a tendency towards acquiescence is more pronounced in placebo reactors. For example, in the study described earlier (page 34) in which a mock physiological recording was used to reinforce the placebo response, the subjects were also asked to complete an acquiescence questionnaire. They were told to indicate with which of a number of statements they agreed. Typical statements were 'Love is the greatest of Arts' and 'Wild colts make good horses'. Subjects who agreed with a large number of the statements, that is those who were highly acquiescent, also reported a significantly greater frequency of side-effects to the placebo.

It is reasonable to ask whether these rather specific traits like suggestibility and acquiescence tell us anything more generally about the personality characteristics of the placebo reactor. Probably not directly in the case of acquiescence which does not seem to be clearly associated with any particular personality type. However, the trait is perhaps slightly more common in people who may be described as somewhat conventional in outlook and who hold rather superficial views from which they are easily swayed. Individuals of this type are perhaps more accepting and less critical of the drug situation than their opposite numbers, the 'nay-sayers', who tend to be more controlled and self-determined.

As for suggestibility, this trait has traditionally been associated with hysteria. This is mainly because of the belief that the hysteric succumbs easily to hypnosis, due to a combination of emotional instability and a basically extraverted personality which makes him very responsive to outside influence. In fact, there is very little evidence for any special connexion between hysteria and suggestibility. Instead, heightened suggestibility appears to be a general characteristic of neuroticism as a whole and does not seem to depend on the basic personality being either introverted or extraverted. Studies of the personalities of placebo reactors tend to support this view. The placebo reactor is consistently neither introverted nor extraverted, though he does more typically show evidence of anxiety and of being more generally neurotic.

Having said this about the influence of personality on the placebo response, it is important to bear in mind the remarks made earlier to the effect that no one personality type can be regarded as a placebo reactor. Other factors in the drug situation itself may be equally, if not more, important in deciding whether a particular individual shows a placebo response. Relationships between personality traits and placebo reaction that are found in one situation may not appear, or may even be reversed, in another situation. This was clearly demonstrated in an important study by Knowles and Lucas [39].

These authors carried out a series of experiments under both 'individual' and 'group' conditions. All the subjects were asked to report on the side-effects of a new psychotropic drug which was, in fact, a small white lactose tablet. Subjects assigned to 'individual' conditions assessed the pill while seated alone in a room. Those assigned to 'group' conditions were seated together in small groups of three. All subjects completed the Maudsley Personality Inventory, a scale giving measures on two personality dimensions, one of extraversion and one of emotional instability, or neuroticism. In two experiments carried out under

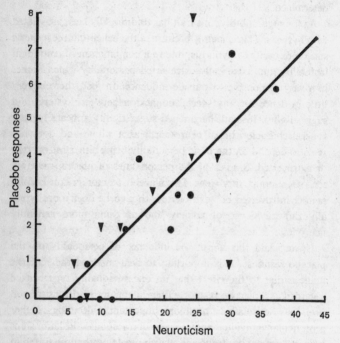

Fig. 2.3. The relationship between placebo reaction and degree of neuroticism. As neuroticism increases so does the number of 'symptoms' reported after taking dummy pills. The results of two experiments are shown separately, the differences between them probably being due to other factors that affect the placebo response (see text). (From a diagram by J. B. Knowles and C. J. Lucas.)

(Reproduced by permission of the authors and the publishers, *Journal of Mental Science.*)

'group' conditions there was a significant positive relationship between neuroticism and the number of placebo side-effects reported. This is illustrated in Figure 2.3 which shows the progressive rise in placebo responses with increasing neuroticism. When a similar comparison was made in two experiments carried out under 'individual' conditions the relationship shown in Figure 2.3 disappeared. In both 'individual' experiments the correlation between neuroticism and frequency of side-effects was almost zero. Neuroticism was therefore only an important determinant of the placebo effect when other, social, influences were also present. When they were absent the presence of a high degree of emotional instability was unimportant. These results confirm the idea that under group conditions of drug administration, as might occur for example in a psychiatric ward, the more suggestible neurotic individual is more likely to 'catch' side-effects from other people around him.

Knowles and Lucas also report some complex relationships with extraversion. In the 'group' experiments there was no overall correlation between placebo response and extraversion, but in one of the 'individual' experiments there was a highly significant tendency for the more extraverted individuals to report more side-effects. However, in the second 'individual' experiment the opposite result was found. There it was the *introverted* subjects who showed the greatest placebo response. The reason for this discrepancy probably lies in the background of the subjects used. The subjects in all of the other experiments were student nurses, whereas in the second 'individual' experiment theological students were employed. Knowles and Lucas suggest that theological students, having little background knowledge of drugs, would report on minor effects which would be disregarded by the more experienced nurses. Introverts would be much more meticulous in doing so, hence the greater placebo response in these personalities.

Finally, in the same investigation Knowles and Lucas also studied the effect of what they termed 'stress' conditions. Most of the subjects carried out their assessment of the placebo in a fairly relaxed situation in which they were simply asked to report on the side-effects they experienced. Some, however, were told that the results would be of crucial importance and that their assessment had to be as accurate as possible. Although these instructions did not alter the relationship between personality and the placebo response, stress did produce overall a significant increase in the number of side-effects reported.

The personality of the placebo reactor, then, is only important in so far as it conditions his response to certain other features that may be present in the drug situation. Characteristics such as suggestibility may come to the fore and produce a high rate of placebo response only if group influences are strongly operating or if the investigator is especially persuasive or if both occur together. Under other conditions different aspects of the personality may take on greater significance. If, for example, the subject is a psychiatric patient and the experiment a therapeutic drug trial, the needs associated with the patient's illness may become of overriding importance. Personality and other factors found to be operative in experiments using normal volunteers may be quite different from those present in drug studies carried out in a hospital setting.

Although the placebo effect is a fascinating curiosity in its own right, it can obviously become a nuisance in drug evaluation studies. Early attempts to discover 'placebo types' were made partly in the hope of being able to eliminate such people from drug experiments. It was thought that if this could be done it would be easier to separate 'real' from 'psychological' drug effects. Since, like so many other psychological reactions, the placebo response is not an all-or-none phenomenon, psychopharmacologists have instead to control for it by careful design of their experiments.

As a therapeutic nostrum the placebo is as old as medicine itself, but as a scientific tool in drug research it is of recent origin. A few workers at the beginning of this century realized the part that suggestion may play in drug effects and designed their experiments to include a control set of observations on subjects given a substitute dummy medication. However, it is only in the past fifteen years or so that the inclusion of a placebo condition has been routine practice in drug studies. The scientific reasons for this precaution will be fairly obvious. As we have seen, the placebo response may be a very powerful one and, even though the psychopharmacologist cannot eliminate it from his experiments, he can try to assess its contribution to the total drug effect that he observes. How this is done is quite simple, at least in principle. Suppose we wish to know whether drug X is having a real pharmacological effect on some piece of behaviour. By taking two sets of measurements, one under the drug and one under an identical placebo, we can determine whether drug X is having an effect over and above that due to the placebo response alone.

There are also growing practical reasons for using placebo controls in drug research. Each year the pharmaceutical industry proliferates its output of new remedies for anxiety, depression, and other psychological ills. It becomes more and more essential to decide whether these panaceas have any greater therapeutic value than the persuasive sugar pill. Many will not and this can only be decided by carefully conducted clinical trials. The basic scientist, as well as the clinician, will have a vested interest in the outcome of such trials. While it is not always true, it very often happens that those drugs which survive as important advances in treatment are also of greatest scientific interest to the research worker who uses drugs to explore the underlying mechanisms of behaviour.

There are legitimate exceptions to the rule of using a dummy placebo as a standard of comparison in drug experiments. We may wish to know whether a particular drug has a different effect from that of another drug whose properties have been well established by previous research. This sometimes happens in clinical drug trials. Supposing drug X has been introduced as a new sedative. It would be reasonable to compare it against one of the well-tried barbiturates which are known from long experience to have strong sedative properties. The definition of a well-tried drug is somewhat arbitrary, of course, and whether the placebo is dispensed with will depend not only on how long the comparison drug has been in use, but also on how much is known about its effect on the particular function being studied. It would be defensible to compare drug X with a barbiturate if we were assessing their relative merits as sleeping pills. If we were studying the effect of drug X on some psychological or physiological measure that had not been investigated before, then a placebo control ought to be used. The barbiturate could still be included, of course, as an additional standard of comparison. This would then involve taking three sets of measurements, one under drug X, one under a placebo and one under an active drug whose general properties were known.

Whether a placebo or another active drug is used for comparison, the design and procedure of the experiment will follow similar lines. The main purpose will be to ensure that all of the measurements are taken under equivalent conditions; so that any differences observed can be put down to the drug or drugs and not to some extraneous factor in the situation. An important requirement will be to eliminate, as far as possible, any bias on the part of the subject or investigator. Where feasible the experiment will be carried out under 'double-blind' conditions. Here neither the subject nor the experimenter will know whether the active drug or the placebo is being used at any particular time. This is achieved by getting someone not involved in the study to assign the 'treatments' randomly according to a code which is only broken at the end of the experiment.

Sometimes the experimenter may have to be content with a single-blind procedure in which only the subject is kept in the dark about what he is given. This often arises where the drug is administered by an injection which for practical reasons must be under the control of the experimenter. In this case the preparation of the subject will be kept the same for both drug and placebo conditions; or the injection procedure may be arranged so that the active solution is unobtrusively substituted for an inert saline solution without the subject being aware of it. Drugs are frequently given by injection in animal experiments and sometimes to human subjects in whom some objective physiological change is being recorded. In these circumstances the observations will be less subject to bias on the part of the experimenter and a single-blind technique will be more acceptable.

Where possible, however, a double-blind procedure will be used and with oral administration the identity of the active drug will be kept secret by making up both the drug and the placebo in pills or capsules of identical size, shape, colour, taste and so on. Alternatively, they may both be administered in liquid form or as a powder disguised in a highly flavoured orange or peppermint drink. Preserving the double-blind may be more difficult than it appears at first sight. Subtle differences in taste or texture may give the subject a clue as to which is the active and which is the inert pill. This can sometimes have quite profound effects on the outcome of the experiment, as the following study illustrates [2].

A trial was carried out to see whether the tranquillizer pecazine would reduce urinary incontinence in chronic psychotic patients. Two matched groups of patients were compared, one being given the drug and the other apparently identical placebo pills. A significant reduction in daytime wetting did occur, but only in the patients receiving placebos. In the drug group there was no change, either in night or daytime wetting. The experimenters concluded that this placebo effect was due to slight differences in the two sets of pills used. Although looking alike, they tasted differently, the placebos being sweet and the drug being rather bitter in taste. This variation in taste probably led to a difference in the attitude with which the patients received their pills. Placebo patients were effectively being given small sweets by the nurses several times a day, whereas patients in the drug group were being given rather unpleasant tasting medicine. The reduced incontinence in the placebo group could therefore be put down to an all-round improvement in the relationship between the nurses and those patients. The outcome of this study is even more surprising if one considers that the subjects were very chronically deteriorated psychotics in whom a strong placebo response would not be expected.

Apart from the physical characteristics of the pills themselves, there are other factors which may cause the double-blind administration of drugs to break down. Most of these occur in therapeutic drug trials carried out in a clinical setting. A typical study would be the comparison of a new antidepressive against a placebo, or a well-used drug of a similar type, such as imipramine. The hospital pharmacist will decide how the various 'treatments', made up in identical capsules, are to be randomly assigned. What the capsules contain will be unknown to the patient, to the nurse who hands them out, and to the psychiatrist who is to rate each patient's improvement. The capsules will be administered chronically at the usual dose of three or four a day for several weeks. During this time it is quite possible that unexpected side-effects will appear in patients on the experimental drug. These will enable all the interested parties concerned to distinguish it from the inert placebo or from the familiar drug. Even if the patient himself does not recognize much difference, the nurses may unwittingly communicate their own opinions to him. Similarly, there will be an unavoidable bias in the psychiatrist's assessment of improvement. Fortunately, these problems are less likely to arise in drug studies of the laboratory type, where single acute doses of drugs are usually given and where the measurements taken are usually more objective.

The use of a placebo control and, where possible, double-blind administration will cut down some of the more obvious sources of bias in drug studies. Adopting these as minimum requirements, the psychopharmacologist then has to decide on a design for his experiment. The simplest plan is to divide the subjects randomly into two groups and give one the drug and the other the placebo. If more than one drug is being studied, then of course the number of groups is increased accordingly. The trouble with this method is that one can never really be sure that the groups are exactly comparable. Any drug effect observed could be due to the groups being different anyway. We could increase the number of subjects used and hope that this would even out any variation between the groups. This would mean testing a very large sample of people, which is not always practicable and not a very efficient way of going about it.

A better way round the problem is to try and match the subjects available on all the characteristics that we think may influence the results. For example, each subject of a particular age is matched against another subject of roughly the same age. Having matched the subjects on all the relevant characteristics the members of each pair are then assigned at random to either the drug or the placebo group. The snag here is knowing which variables can be safely ignored. If too many are included it may be difficult, if not impossible, to find people who are exactly matched on all of them. In most psychological studies it is usually considered adequate if the subjects are matched for age, sex and some relevant personality characteristic.

A safeguard that sometimes helps is also to match people on the measure that is to be studied in the experiment itself. Supposing we were interested in the effect of a particular drug on simple reaction time. Before carrying out the experiment proper we could give each subject a short run-through on the apparatus and establish a set of baseline reaction times which could then be used for matching purposes. This method is only useful, however, if the measure being studied is fairly stable over time and if we do not mind the subject getting prior experience of the experimental situation. For example, it would be of no value – indeed it would ruin the experiment – if we were intending to study the effect of a drug on the learning of a new task.

An alternative to using separate drug and placebo groups, and hoping that they will be comparable, is to give both 'treatments' to every subject. In this way there will be no matching problems because each subject will, as it were, be matched against himself and so act as his own control. A direct comparison can then be made between each subject's performance while on the drug with his performance while on the placebo. With this design it is necessary to balance the order in which the 'treatments' are given. If all the subjects had the placebo first and then the drug we could not conclude very much even if we found they had different effects. The subjects might have changed in any case from one occasion to the next. What is done instead is to divide the group into two equal halves. Subjects in one half are given the placebo followed by the drug; those in the other half receive the drug first and then the placebo. More complicated designs of a similar type make it possible to administer a number of drugs in a balanced order.

Even this 'cross-over' design, as it is called, is not perfect. Subjects given the drug first might experience effects that carry over to the placebo condition. This may boost their placebo response relative to that of subjects in the other half of the group who receive the placebo without any prior experience of the active drug. The fact that identical pills are used throughout will not help matters because the subjects will naturally assume that they have been given the same thing on both occasions. The carry-over effect is not so great if the subject is made to feel that different pills are being used in the two halves of the experiment. This can be achieved by using pills of different colours, as was done in an experiment carried out recently in our own department [16]. Medical students were asked to report any feelings of sedation they experienced after taking capsules containing either the barbiturate, amobarbital, or a lactose placebo. The capsules were coloured either white or yellow and, in order to preserve the double-blind, both the active drug and the placebo were made up in each of these colours. The students were tested on two occasions, a week apart, some having 'yellow drug' followed by 'yellow placebo', others 'white drug' then 'yellow placebo' and so on. As expected, a high proportion of those who had the active drug first (either white or yellow) reported that they felt sedated. In some subjects this effect carried over to the following week when they were given placebos. The carry-over effect was much greater, however, in those subjects who were given a placebo capsule of the same colour as that used the previous week for the active drug. Eighty-two per cent of the students said they felt sedated after receiving an identical placebo; whereas only eighteen per cent reported any symptoms when their second capsule was switched to a different colour. The frequency with which symptoms were reported was not affected by colour as such, which simply drew the subjects' attention to the fact that different drugs were probably being used in the experiment. Each capsule could then be assessed on its own merits.

The method used in this study of overcoming the carry-over effect is rather cumbersome because it means making up four different preparations of the drug and placebo. It also makes the experimental design rather intricate if the contents and colour of the capsules are to be permutated in a balanced order. For most purposes this is probably carrying the double-blind procedure a bit too far. A similar result can be achieved more easily by just being honest with the subject and informing him that different drugs, or a drug and a placebo, will be used during the experiment. He can be told that the capsules only look alike because neither he nor the experimenter is supposed to know which is which. He may not believe this, of course, but then the research worker cannot have it all ways!

Although no experimental design can be perfect, in practice most of the extraneous factors that can affect drug response tend to cancel themselves out; assuming, of course, that the experiment has been well planned in the first place and most of the obvious biases have been eliminated. The point is that the effects of a powerful drug will still show, despite the placebo response. If they do not show, then the action of the drug is probably not of

much significance anyway. In the following chapters we shall
return to the main theme of the book and look at some of the
ways in which drugs, acting as drugs, help to bring behaviour
under experimental control.

Drugs, Wakefulness and Sleep 3

Two chapters ago I mentioned some of the drugs that you, the reader, may have taken before picking up this book. Those of you who drank some strong black coffee with the intention of 'knocking off' the book in an evening are probably still with us. Those who combine their bedtime reading with a sleeping pill are probably not and have doubtless reached this point several – I trust well-rested – nights later. In both cases the drugs concerned will have had roughly opposite effects. Caffeine in the coffee will have made you a little more alert and helped ward off the effects of fatigue. The sleeping pill will have relaxed you and accentuated the restful effects of warmth and quiet. These changes in wakefulness are among the most familiar effects of the commoner psychotropic drugs, especially those classified as stimulant or sedative. This feature of their action is best understood if one considers how even under natural conditions, when we have not taken drugs, our level of consciousness fluctuates over time. Quite apart from the eight or so hours spent asleep at night, there is a constant rise and fall in the daytime waking state which is influenced by many factors, both inside and outside the organism. At certain times of the day we may be more alert than at others, a diurnal rhythm that is probably independent of what we are doing. On the other hand, if things around us get too monotonous we may find ourselves dozing, however wide-awake and attentive we were to begin with. Other situations may make demands upon us that keep us on our toes, like the live broadcaster waiting for his cue. Just occasionally under certain circumstances we may become so aroused that the excitement leads to a panic state.

These fluctuations in conscious awareness are not discrete steps but represent a continuously variable state from sleep at one end to extreme panic at the other. The major stimulant and sedative drugs can be thought of as an artificial means of pushing the individual up or down this continuum, as shown in Figure 3.1. Thus, the stimulant drugs, like the amphetamine group, will

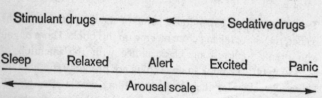

Fig. 3.1. The sleep-wake or arousal scale, illustrating the opposite effects produced by stimulant and sedative drugs.

tend to shift the individual towards a state of higher arousal; while sedatives, such as the barbiturates, will shift him in the opposite direction and, if given in large enough doses, will induce a state of deep anaesthesia. Needless to say, there are a number of complications to this very simple view of drug action, especially when we come to try and explain the effects of some of the newer psychotropic drugs. For the moment, however, it provides a useful working model for understanding some of the drug effects to be described in this chapter.

One way of demonstrating the effect of psychotropic drugs on this sleep-wake continuum would be to administer graded doses of two drugs, a stimulant and a sedative, and ask people to rate their subjective feelings of alertness or drowsiness. Alternatively, the experimenter himself could rate the subjects' overt behaviour. In either case increasing dosage of the drugs would be accompanied by increasing signs of upward or downward shifts in wakefulness. A better way of doing the same thing is to study the more subtle physiological changes that occur as the individual's arousal level varies, either naturally or under drugs. Many of these changes are controlled by the autonomic nervous system which is responsible for such involuntary responses as the slowing of the heart during sleep or relaxation and its sudden acceleration during high excitement. Changes along the continuum shown in Figure 3.1 are, in fact, accompanied by a complex pattern of autonomic reactions, but one of the most sensitive is the variation in sweat gland activity. This can be fairly easily measured by passing a very tiny current through an electrode attached to a part of the skin that is rich in sweat glands, such as the palms of the hands or the soles of the feet. The ease with which the current flows through the skin will vary with the amount of sweat secreted under the electrode so that minute changes in sweating can be recorded as electrical signals on a meter or moving chart. (In practice, the changes are recorded as a variation in resistance to the current and then converted to a measure of conductance.)

The general level of conductance varies with our state of alertness, gradually decreasing as sweat gland activity falls during sleep and increasing when we awake. In addition to this rather slow drift in skin conductance other abrupt changes occur from time to time. These discrete reactions, known as galvanic skin responses or GSRs, appear if we are suddenly stimulated, especially if we are startled by, say, a loud noise. Sometimes,

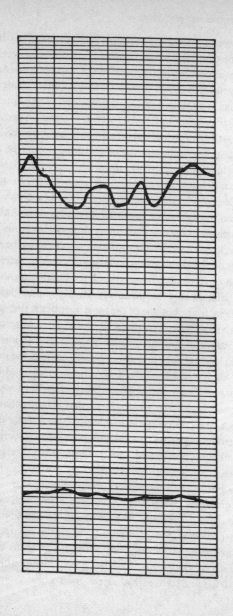

however, they occur for no apparent reason even when there is no obvious variation in the surroundings. These spontaneous GSRs, as they are called, appear to reflect the internal state of the individual; being very numerous during emotional excitement and often disappearing altogether when we are relaxed.

Changes in sweat gland activity, especially the number of spontaneous GSRs, provide a convenient way of monitoring the effect of drugs on the level of alertness. A simple example of this is illustrated in Figure 3.2, which shows how an injection of the barbiturate, amobarbital, can completely eliminate spontaneous GSR activity. While he was waiting for the injection the subject was naturally fairly nervous and so spontaneous GSRs were quite frequent (upper tracing). During the injection these gradually reduced in number until, after a dosage sufficient to make the subject drowsy, they disappeared altogether (lower tracing).

Two American workers, Burch and Greiner, have used this procedure to quantify changes along the sleep-wake continuum when subjects are given different doses of stimulant and sedative drugs [9]. To study sedative effects they used another barbiturate, thiopental, which is similar to but acts for a shorter time than amobarbital. The stimulant drug they used was pentetrazol which has a strongly excitant action on the nervous system. Burch and Greiner injected each of these drugs and counted the number of spontaneous skin responses per minute that occurred at several dose levels. As expected, they found that with increasing dose the frequency of GSRs gradually fell under thiopental and gradually rose under pentetrazol. By combining the results for a number of subjects they were able to reconstruct the whole spectrum of arousal from sleep to excitement. This is illustrated in Figure 3.3,

Fig. 3.2. Example of the effects of the sedative, amobarbital, on the frequency of spontaneous galvanic skin responses. Upper tracing was recorded just before administration of the drug and shows frequent changes in skin resistance in an alert and slightly anxious subject. Lower tracing was taken from the same subject a few minutes later, after injection of enough drug to make him drowsy. At this point spontaneous GSRs have almost entirely disappeared.

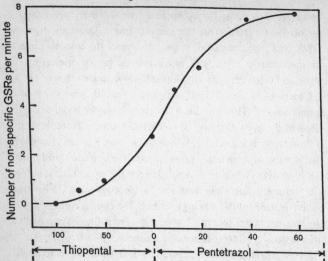

Fig. 3.3. Effect of two drugs, thiopental sodium and pentetrazol, on level of arousal as measured by the frequency of spontaneous or non-specific galvanic skin responses. Each point represents the average for a number of subjects. Note the steady change in GSR frequency with increasing dose of sedative (to the left) and stimulant (to the right).

(Reproduced by permission of N. R. Burch and T. H. Greiner and of the American Psychiatric Association.)

which clearly shows the progressive change in GSR frequency as the two drugs exerted an increasingly stimulant or sedative action.

One familiar consequence of an upward or downward shift in alertness is that the ability to perform various tasks may improve or deteriorate. As with the physiological changes just described, so performance will fluctuate due to fatigue or excitement. Again these natural variations can be simulated by giving the subject a drug which it is known will make him more or less alert. The change in his performance can then be measured and related to the dose administered. Generally speaking the

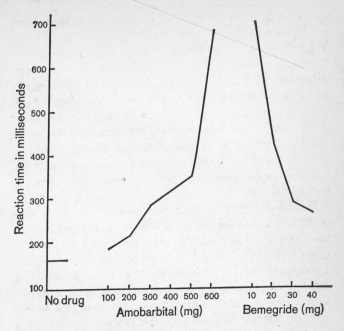

Fig. 3.4. Effects of injecting two drugs on the reaction time of a single subject. With increasing dose of amobarbital reaction time gets steadily longer. An injection of the stimulant bemegride given immediately afterwards reverses the effect and reaction time gradually gets quicker again. Each point represents the mean of four reaction times measured at fifteen-second intervals during the injections.

larger the dose the more performance will be affected. This is most clearly demonstrated by giving the drug as a slow injection and taking frequent measurements of some simple response, like reaction time. Figure 3.4 shows the result of one such experiment carried out in our own laboratory. First of all, sedative effects were produced with a slow continuous injection of amobarbital. Reaction time was measured by having the subject rest his free hand on a metal plate with his middle finger in contact with a round metal button. Four times a minute, roughly every fifteen

seconds, a shock was delivered through the button. The subject
was instructed to lift his finger as quickly as possible whenever
he felt the shock, the speed of his reaction being measured by a
timer incorporated in the circuit. Figure 3.4 illustrates how,
compared with a series of readings taken before any drug was
given, the subject's reactions became progressively longer as he
became more and more sedated. Immediately following this part
of the experiment a stimulant drug, bemegride, was injected. It
can be seen that during this phase reaction times gradually
speeded up again as the subject became more awake; although
with the dose of drug administered they never quite returned to
normal.

There is an obvious similarity between these results and those
of Burch and Greiner. Sedation reduces physiological activity
and slows down performance, while stimulant drugs have the
opposite effect of alerting the subject and speeding up reactions.
Unfortunately the story does not end here. Although over a wide
range of the sleep-wake continuum performance and physiological arousal change roughly in parallel, they tend to part
company when arousal gets very high. Beyond a certain critical
point increasing excitement actually causes performance to
deteriorate, so that the more aroused we get the more our
performance is disrupted. This is why tranquillizers, which have
a mild sedative action, both calm us and help us to concentrate on
a difficult task.

We can see how this comes about if we look at Figure 3.5,
which illustrates how physiological arousal and performance are
related. It is clear from this diagram that under some circumstances sedative drugs will actually *improve* performance, rather
than make it worse. Suppose, for example, that we have a subject
who is so highly anxious that he is placed somewhere towards the
extreme right end of the dotted line representing the arousal
scale. His corresponding position on the bell-shaped curve representing performance will be well below that of peak efficiency. It
follows that a sedative drug should, as it were, push the subject

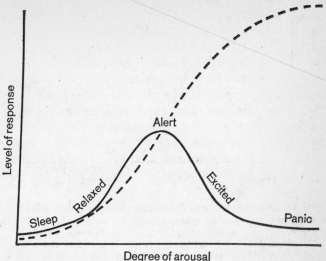

Fig. 3.5. Diagram illustrating how physiological response (dotted line) and overt behaviour (solid line) alter as arousal level changes. Note the tendency for behaviour to become less efficient as physiological arousal increases beyond an optimum point and the mental states of excitement and panic supervene.

(Reproduced by permission of N. R. Burch and T. H. Greiner and of the American Psychiatric Association.)

to the left towards the 'alert' position, reducing his physiological arousal but improving his performance. Of course, if further amounts of drug are given and he is pushed beyond the optimum point, both performance and arousal will once more decline together.

How does this work out in practice? Figure 3.6 shows the results of another of our own experiments which illustrates the effect just described. The subject was a highly anxious neurotic patient taking part in a reaction time study similar to that described earlier. However, in this case we gave only the sedative drug (amobarbital) and instead of measuring reaction time to an

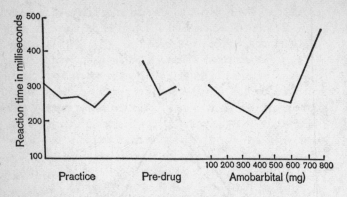

Fig. 3.6. Effect of amobarbital on the reaction time of a very anxious man; illustrating how, during the early part of the injection, his performance actually improved as the drug made him more relaxed. Note particularly how even under a relatively large dose of sedative this subject's responses were quicker than before the injection was begun. Each point represents the mean of four reaction times recorded at fifteen-second intervals throughout the experiment.

electric shock, a loud buzzer was used as the stimulus. The drug was again administered as a slow continuous injection, and reaction times measured every fifteen seconds or so. Just before the experiment proper a series of reaction times was taken to establish a baseline and put the subject at his ease. The hypodermic needle was then inserted and a few more practice trials were given. As can be seen in the diagram, at the beginning of this pre-drug phase the subject's performance was severely disrupted, presumably by anxiety about the injection procedure. Once performance had returned to normal the injection was started. It can be seen that during this period the subject's reaction times became steadily faster up to an optimum level and then began to slow down as the increasing dose of drug took him beyond the peak of the performance curve. Unfortunately, we did not have an independent measure of the patient's physiological state during the experiment, but if we had counted, say, spontaneous GSRs we would have expected him to show a very high rate at the beginning and a slower decline under the drug than a less anxious person.

This experiment also illustrates the enormous variability in individual tolerance of drugs. The extent of the variation can be seen if we compare the response of our neurotic patient with that of the normal subject who took part in the similar reaction time experiment described earlier. As can be seen in Figure 3.6, the second subject was still responding quite well after 600 mg. of the drug had been injected. In fact, his performance at this point was slightly better than his average reaction time before the experiment started. A look back at Figure 3.4 on page 57 shows that after a similar amount of drug had been injected the first subject was so sleepy that he was scarcely able to respond at all. Later in the book I shall have more to say about the reasons for these individual differences in drug tolerance.

The experiments described so far have all been concerned with the immediate effects of drugs administered progressively by injection, sometimes up to quite high doses, and have involved studying how a simple response changes over a relatively short period of time. As we have seen, this method is a useful way of exploring the full spectrum of drug effects in a single individual. Drugs injected directly into the blood-stream have a rapid action on the brain, giving the experimenter precise control over his subjects' level of arousal. Within a few minutes he can cover a wide range of responsiveness.

Interest in the general effect of drugs on wakefulness and attention has, however, led to a series of experiments of a slightly different kind. These have used small doses of drugs to manipulate behaviour in people performing tasks that require prolonged attention. We saw earlier that shifts along the sleep-wake continuum are a natural feature of nervous activity, which is in a continuous state of flux due to changes in the brain's own biological rhythm and in the external influences to which it is exposed. Above all, the brain dislikes monotony and in order to

maintain it at an adequate level of alertness it requires a constantly varying input of stimuli. Normally it gets this but occasionally it meets a situation where its vigilance falters and brief
or more prolonged drops in physiological arousal occur. This
is especially likely under certain environmental conditions that
most of us have experienced. The long drive up a deserted motorway or the drone of a dry lecture are familiar situations in which
the drift towards sleep may make us dangerously (or embarras-
singly!) incapable of dealing with any sudden demands that are
made upon us.

The fluctuating nature of human attention became of practical
concern during the Second World War when it was discovered
that operators keeping an extended watch on radar screens
occasionally failed to detect vital information. Subsequent experiments by N. H. Mackworth revealed that these lapses of
attention were a characteristic feature of tasks of this kind,
especially at the end of a long watch. The task Mackworth used
was not radar-watching itself but involved a clock with a pointer
that made regular discrete jumps. From time to time at random
intervals the pointer would make a double jump which formed the
'signals' to be detected by the operator. Various ways of preventing decline in performance on this task were described,
including the use of drugs. It was found, for example, that if the
subjects were given amphetamine they missed fewer signals than
if they performed without the drug.

Since Mackworth carried out these experiments other studies
have demonstrated similar effects of drugs on the performance
of a variety of vigilance tasks, as they are sometimes called. A
recent experiment compared the effect of a drug of the amphetamine group, methamphetamine, with that of a sedative, pentobarbital [68]. All the subjects taking part received both drugs and
a saline control injection, administered in a balanced order.
After each treatment they performed for one hour on a task of
visual search. This involved watching a continuously changing
pattern of lights, each of which showed a digit flashing on and off

at irregular intervals. The number of digits showing at any one time could vary up to a maximum of nine. The subject was required to watch out for the number '4' and to press a key whenever it occurred. Figure 3.7 shows the main results of this experiment. Compared with the saline condition, pentobarbital significantly reduced the number of 'signals' detected, while methamphetamine had the opposite effect of increasing the efficiency of performance.

Apart from lowering or raising the general level of alertness, precisely how do these drug effects come about? We now know that performance on repetitive tasks of this kind does not proceed uniformly. Instead, it is punctuated by a series of brief involuntary rest pauses, lasting a second or two, when the subject takes time off from the task in order to recuperate. These 'microsleeps', as they have also been called, are noticed subjectively as lapses of attention, often followed by a brief period of feeling more than usually wide awake: an experience familiar to hardened lecture-goers! Objectively they appear in performance as blocks or gaps when no response is made. The exact physiological basis of these pauses is unknown, but their onset is probably due to the gradual accumulation, in the nervous system, of an inhibitory process which the pause allows to be dissipated. If an EEG recording is taken during their occurrence, it is found that brain activity shows characteristic signs of sleep.

Involuntary rest pauses are more likely to occur in states of low arousal and one way in which sedative drugs probably impair performance on vigilance tasks is by increasing the likelihood of rest pauses occurring. If the subject is taking frequent rest pauses, there is a high probability that some of them will coincide with a 'signal' which he is supposed to detect but which he will inevitably miss. His overall performance will therefore be reduced. Stimulant drugs, on the other hand, delay the onset of rest pauses and increase the chances that the subject is paying attention when a 'signal' occurs. Testing this idea with ordinary vigilance tasks is not too easy, because we do not have a

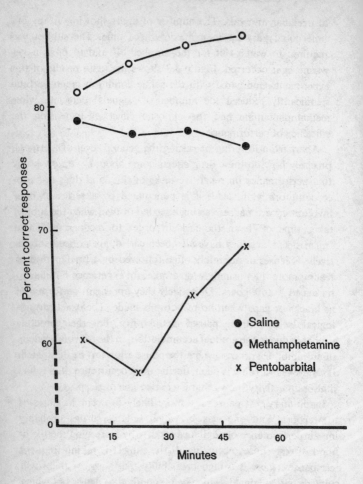

Fig. 3.7. Effect of two drugs and a saline placebo on the performance of a vigilance task, showing the average number of 'signals' detected in each fifteen minutes of a one-hour watch. (From a diagram by G. A. Talland and G. C. Quarton).

(Reproduced by permission of the authors and the publishers, *Journal of Nervous and Mental Disease*.)

continuous measure of the subject's behaviour. Most of the time he is just sitting in front of a display waiting for something to happen and it is difficult, if not impossible, to detect gaps in his performance. Fortunately, there are other types of task which show similar characteristics and on which signs of blocking can be measured. These tasks require the subject to make repetitive responses which are usually so simple that practice effects do not complicate the issue and which allow his behaviour to be monitored continuously. A favourite example is the serial reaction time task described in the previous chapter. Here, it will be recalled, the subject has continually to press the correct one of a series of keys in order to extinguish a light and illuminate another light to which a further response is made and so on. Arranged in this way the task is self-paced, that is to say the subject can perform as quickly or as slowly as he wishes, depending on how rapidly he keeps up the cycle of light-off and light-on. Performance is normally characterized by a steady rate of responding as each light comes on, with an occasional reaction time that is longer than usual. These involuntary rests are frequently accompanied by an error in which the wrong key is selected. This temporarily blocks performance until the subject recovers and presses the right key in order to start the performance cycle again. A measure of the errors committed therefore provides a good index of the number of involuntary rest pauses occurring on the test.

Dr Herrington in our own department recently examined the effects of amphetamine on this task [29]. He tested three groups of medical students randomly assigned to drug, no drug, and placebo conditions. The students performed for ten minutes on a typical serial reaction time apparatus consisting of four lights, each with a corresponding key. To his surprise the drug had absolutely no effect on the overall rate of response on the test, all three groups performing at exactly the same level throughout the ten minutes. However, as illustrated in Figure 3.8 the number of errors committed under amphetamine was markedly lower than under

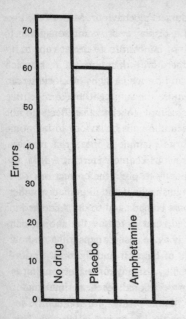

Fig. 3.8. A comparison of the mean error scores of three groups of subjects carrying out a continuous reaction time task under different conditions. Note the marked reduction in errors committed by subjects performing on amphetamine.

(Permission to report these results was kindly given by R. N. Herrington.)

either of the other two treatment conditions. Dr Herrington concluded that the main effect of amphetamine was to reduce the subject's need to take frequent rest pauses during performance.

Before leaving this topic it may interest some readers to know that another drug consumed daily by many people, namely nicotine, also has arousing properties and, like amphetamine, has been found to delay the onset of rest pauses on repetitive tasks. This may surprise those for whom the soothing weed is a cure in any crisis. In fact, nicotine has no sedative properties but is a potent stimulant of the autonomic and central nervous systems; included among its effects being the release of epinephrine into the blood-stream. Of course, we all know that there is more to smoking than just nicotine and its apparently calming influence is probably due to other incidental factors associated with the habit, such as deep inhaling or satisfying a primitive oral need. However, it is also claimed that smoking helps concentration on a difficult task. This is probably due to the stimulating action of nicotine itself which, in the way I have described, will help to sustain attention by offsetting the effects of mental fatigue.

Changing the frequency with which it takes a rest is one way, then, in which the brain reacts to shifts in its arousal level, whether this is induced by drugs or by the external environment, or by both. Normally these rest pauses only become a nuisance under rather special conditions of extreme monotony and even then only after sufficient time has elapsed for a rest pause to become necessary. There is, however, another more immediate way in which our attention to the environment is altered in different states of physiological arousal. As arousal level rises the number and range of stimuli to which we pay attention diminishes; or, put another way, we become less distracted by stimuli that are not our immediate concern. This mechanism obviously serves a useful biological purpose. In emergencies, for example, the organism can take much more effective action if irrelevant features of the environment are screened out and attention is focussed only on those that are important to the job in hand. Which stimuli are selected will depend upon the situation in which arousal occurs. The surprised lover intent upon escape hardly needs to take in the colour of the irate husband's eyes.

This idea that the span of attention narrows or broadens as the general level of arousal rises or falls has been the subject of a number of laboratory experiments, particularly by an American worker, Callaway, who has used various procedures to demonstrate the effect [10]. One way has been to study how changes in arousal level affect a common perceptual phenomenon, that of size-constancy. The latter refers to the fact that in perceiving the size of objects we always correct for the distance they are away from us. For example, a penny viewed from the other side of the room will still look larger than a sixpence held in the hand even though the image it projects on the retina will actually be smaller. One reason we can make this correction is that we normally rely on help from other visual cues in the environment. It has been argued, therefore, that people who are made highly aroused will correct less than they should for distance because their narrowed attention will prevent them using as many surrounding cues as they otherwise would. Consequently, distant objects will appear relatively smaller than usual. Callaway tested out this hypothesis by getting subjects to match the size of a square patch of light projected on a distant screen with a standard square placed immediately in front of them. He found that arousing them in various ways, including giving them the drug methamphetamine, caused them to under-correct for distance and make the far square smaller than they did under control conditions. Of course, even on the drug the subjects showed a good deal of size-constancy, but relatively speaking it was less than normal; thus supporting the idea that changes in arousal will alter the range of stimuli attended to during perceptual judgements.

Variations in the breadth of attention probably play an important part in many kinds of human performance, including performance on some of the other tasks described earlier. Detection of signals on the vigilance type of task, for example, will be better if the individual is not distracted by incidental features of the visual display. This is another way, therefore, in which stimulant drugs help to maintain a high rate of signal detection. Of course, attention that is too narrowed will be a positive disadvantage on some tasks where constant scanning of the environment is called for. It is all a matter of degree and, as is the case with most psychological functions, there will be an optimum level that is different for each task.

We have, then, seen several important ways in which drugs can alter the organism's responsiveness to its environment. They can shift its general level of alertness as well as improve or interfere with the ability to select certain stimuli and reject others. At the same time drugs can increase or decrease resistance to the mental fatigue or inhibition that is a characteristic of brain function under certain conditions. Each of these changes is almost certainly controlled by a different mechanism in the nervous system but, because everything there is usually nicely integrated, under normal circumstances they will all tend to work together. Thus, the individual whose arousal level is shifted upwards will become generally more alert, will show narrowing of attention, and will be less affected by monotony. The experimenter can to some extent disentangle these various effects in the laboratory by designing tests that throw up one kind of change rather than another. Measuring changes in size-constancy, for example, may be quite a good way of determining how drugs alter the breadth of attention. It is clearly of little use, however, for studying the effect of drugs on work decrement, where vigilance and continuous performance tasks are more suitable.

Another way of tackling the same problem is to compare other drugs that are thought to have more specific effects on the brain than ordinary stimulants and sedatives, which tend to produce rather global changes. So far I have confined myself to these two drug groups because the marked contrast between them helps to bring out some of the fundamental principles of drug action. Some of the newer psychotropic drugs, however, do not fit too well into this simple model. The tranquillizers are a good example. These drugs are sedative up to a point and, like barbiturates, they reduce GSR activity and slow down performance. The effects are not quite so marked, however, at least when they are given in normal doses. Subjectively, there is a difference too. Tranquillizers calm you down without producing that 'woolly' feeling complained about after taking drugs like phenobarbital and amobarbital. Psychopharmacologists can put this selective action of drugs to good use by comparing how different bits of behaviour are affected by different drugs. In this way they can build up a kind of profile of each drug's effect and at the same time hope to discover something more about the underlying mechanisms of behaviour. This use of drugs is still in its infancy, especially in human psychopharmacology, but a couple of examples will help to illustrate the point being made.

The first example is taken from the work of a group of American scientists who have compared the effects of different tranquillizers and sedatives on various speed and sustained attention tasks [47]. As expected, the general effect of both types of drug was to depress performance. Relative to each other, however, the drugs had different effects depending on the kind of performance change measured. One comparison they made was between the major tranquillizer, chlorpromazine, and two sedatives, secobarbital and phenobarbital. The performance of subjects given these drugs was compared on two tasks. One was a digit-symbol test in which the subject was required to write symbols underneath rows of digits according to a predetermined code. The other was what they called the Continuous Performance Test, or CPT. Here the subject had to watch a continuous display on which letters appeared one at a time in a random order. His job was to press a key whenever he saw the letter A appear followed immediately by the letter X. Compared with placebo conditions, performance of both tests was worse under all three drug treatments, but the *relative* effect of the drugs was different. As shown in Figure 3.9, chlorpromazine had a much greater effect on CPT performance than it did on the digit-symbol test. Its effects were similar to those of sleep deprivation which, for interest's sake, are also shown in the diagram. The results for the two sedative drugs were quite opposite to this. Both of these drugs impaired digit-symbol performance but had relatively less effect on the CPT. These findings can probably be explained by the fact that the two tests measure different things and were therefore picking up differences in the action of the two types of drug. The

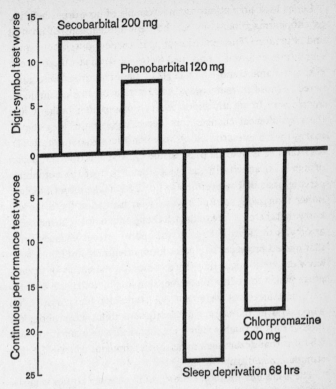

Fig. 3.9. Diagram showing the relative effects of different drugs on two psychological tasks, described in detail in the text. Points to notice are the difference between the two barbiturate drugs and chlorpromazine and the latter's similarity to a period of sleep deprivation.

(Diagram by A. F. Mirsky and H. E. Rosvold, reproduced by their permission and that of Messrs. John Wiley and Sons, Inc.)

digit-symbol test is a fairly simple speed task which would be easily affected by the globally depressant action of sedative drugs. The Continuous Performance Test, on the other hand, is more sensitive to momentary fluctuations in attention, which is thought to be especially affected by chorpromazine and similar drugs.

Let us look now at our second example of how drugs help the psychopharmacologist dissect the basic mechanisms of arousal and attention. This experiment was carried out in our own laboratory and was concerned with the comparison between dexamphetamine and LSD-25 [14]. These two drugs were compared because in many ways LSD acts a bit like a stimulant. People very frequently report feeling anxious after taking it and the physiological changes that occur support the idea that it makes them more aroused. A very consistent response to LSD, for example, is that the pupil of the eye gets much larger, a sign of increased activity in the sympathetic part of the autonomic nervous system. The overall effect of LSD is therefore stimulant rather than sedative. But anyone who has taken the drug will know that there is more to the LSD effect than this. The increased anxiety is the least part of it, the more obvious changes being that mental processes like perception, attention, and thinking go haywire. We thought that if we compared the effects of dexamphetamine and LSD on some simple physiological and behavioural measures we might get some clue about how LSD works and at the same time learn something more about the mechanisms through which it acts. Basically we wanted to know why it is that dexamphetamine is just stimulant whereas LSD is stimulant *and* disruptive.

The measures we took were carefully chosen to tap what we felt were the important physiological and psychological functions that were affected by the two drugs. One was a measure of simple reaction time, where the subject had to respond as quickly as possible to a light coming on. A second was a measure called the two-flash threshold test. Here the subject is shown a pair of brief flashes of light with a very short interval between them, measured in milliseconds. This interval is reduced until the light flashes fuse and they appear subjectively as one light. Usually a second set of readings is also taken, starting with what appears to be a single light and increasing the interval until the subject says he can detect two flashes. The two-flash threshold is the point of change-over from one subjective impression to the other. Since the two ways of finding the threshold often give slightly different results, the measures obtained are usually averaged. Normally, as arousal level increases, discrimination on this test gets better, that is, the interval at which the subject can still see two flashes gets shorter.

Reaction time and two-flash threshold were measured at regular intervals for two hours after each drug had been administered. The subjects were actually tested on three occasions because a placebo condition was also included, with each subject acting as his own control. Throughout each two-hour testing session the subject was hooked up to a polygraphic recording device which continuously monitored various types of physiological activity. The one I want to mention here is skin potential, which we have already come across in a slightly different form, namely skin conductance. Skin potential is like skin conductance in that it also reflects sweat-gland response, but instead of passing a current and measuring the resistance to it the actual electrical activity of the skin is amplified and recorded.

What effects did we expect the two drugs to have on these different measures? We thought that dexamphetamine would have a fairly uniform effect, increasing physiological arousal, improving discrimination on the two-flash threshold test, and speeding up reaction time. Frankly, we did not know what to expect with LSD, though we thought that physiological arousal would increase in much the same way as with dexamphetamine. Figure 3.10 illustrates the drug effects that occurred during the first hour of testing. After that time the changes were difficult to interpret and in any case they were a bit unreliable, at least when the subjects were on LSD. By the second hour they were either enjoying their model psychoses or wishing they had not taken the stuff. In neither case were they too cooperative about doing our silly tests!

A look at Figure 3.10 shows that dexamphetamine had the sort of effect we had predicted, all of the measures showing evidence of a generally upward shift in arousal. Compared with

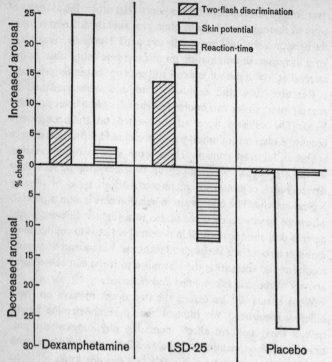

Fig. 3.10. Diagram illustrating differences in the 'profiles' of effects produced on three measures by dexamphetamine, LSD-25, and a placebo. Upward bars represent changes indicative of increased arousal, i.e. raised skin potential, improved two-flash discrimination, and quicker reaction time. Downward bars indicate the opposite. Note the uniform, though opposite, effects of dexamphetamine and placebo and the more complex action of LSD, particularly its relatively greater effect on two-flash discrimination compared with dexamphetamine (see text for further explanation).

placebo conditions, where arousal went down as the subject became used to the situation, dexamphetamine increased skin potential, improved two-flash discrimination, and shortened the reaction time. The effects of LSD were more complicated. As expected, physiological arousal increased, but rather less than with dexamphetamine. On the other hand, perceptual discrimination on the two-flash threshold test improved considerably – over twice as much as on dexamphetamine. The most marked effect of LSD, however, was on reaction time which became steadily slower and slower. Our interpretation of these results was that, unlike the global arousing effects of dexamphetamine, LSD appeared to have a special action on perceptual mechanisms, increasing the individual's sensitivity to stimuli in his environment. The slowing of reaction that occurred was probably due to the fact that the light the subject was supposed to respond to was only one of numerous other curious stimuli that he was trying to cope with at the same time.

The two studies just described were chosen deliberately because in contrasting ways they illustrate a similar point, namely that both chlorpromazine and LSD-25 appear to have a selective effect on certain aspects of arousal, principally those to do with how we react to stimuli in the external environment. As we shall see in a later chapter (Chapter Eight), some psychopharmacologists believe that, unlike sedatives and stimulants, drugs like chlorpromazine and LSD do not alter the level of consciousness as such but have a special action on the brain mechanisms controlling the filtering or screening of stimuli that are allowed to reach consciousness. Is this the same thing as the broadening and narrowing of attention that we have come across before? The answer is probably 'yes' and this is why hallucinogens and the major tranquillizers particularly affect performance on tasks where focussing of attention is important. They act in opposite directions, of course, and it is no coincidence that chlorpromazine is used to treat schizophrenia which, like LSD psychosis, is characterized by gross disorder of attention. For the scientist the selective action of these two drug groups is very convenient because it helps him sort out influences on behaviour that are normally difficult to disentangle.

By now the reader must be having fairly frequent involuntary rest pauses so let us finish this chapter with a few words about drugs in relation to sleep. As we saw earlier, any sedative given in a sufficiently large dose will induce a state of deep sleep, whether the individual likes it or not. Few people receive sedatives in such a quantity unless they are given them as an anaesthetic in preparation for some medical or surgical treatment. An alarming number of people, on the other hand, take them in smaller doses as sleeping pills. In order to escape from their worries during the day-time too, a large number of people also take a variety of other pills, such as tranquillizers and anti-depressive drugs. We have already seen what effect some of these drugs have on behaviour during our waking hours. What effect do they have during the equally important third of our lives spent asleep?

Some study of this topic has been carried out by Dr Ian Oswald and his colleagues in the Edinburgh Department of Psychiatry. They, and other workers elsewhere, have found that many commonly used drugs affect the sleep pattern, mainly by changing the *type* of sleep people get. It is now agreed that there are two main kinds of sleep, orthodox sleep and so-called paradoxical sleep, which differ in a number of important ways. One way of distinguishing between them is by means of the electro-encephalogram. During orthodox sleep the brain waves are large and slow, exactly as would be expected in the state of low arousal associated with sleep. During paradoxical sleep, on the other hand, the brain waves are much smaller and of faster frequency, more like one finds in people who are awake and very alert. This is particularly odd because in some ways it seems to be a deeper form of sleep, as shown by the fact that the muscles are much more relaxed than during orthodox sleep. Paradoxical sleep has also been called dream or rapid-eye-movement (REM) sleep. This is because dreaming occurs mainly during the paradoxical phase and is accompanied by rapid movements of the eyes, almost as though the person were 'watching' the scene he is dreaming.

On average the normal person spends about a quarter of the

night in paradoxical sleep but this pattern may be considerably altered by drugs. Dr Oswald has shown that a single dose of sedative can reduce the proportion of the night spent in REM sleep from the usual twenty-five per cent to nearly five per cent [48]. If sleeping pills have been used regularly and they are then suddenly withdrawn the person spends a few nights when the amount of REM sleep is greater than usual; trying to catch up, as it were, on his lost dreaming time. Curiously enough amphetamine, and the notorious 'purple hearts' mixture of dexamphetamine and amobarbital, also reduce paradoxical sleep; thus apparently contradicting the idea that the effect of amphetamine is opposite to that of the sedatives. Maybe the reason for this paradoxical effect of amphetamine during sleep is that, unlike sedatives, it is normally taken in the day-time in order to stay awake. Perhaps the individual's dream mechanisms are well stimulated during the day and he has less need to use up dream time when he finally gets to sleep; a kind of rebound effect in reverse.

What about other drugs, such as tranquillizers? The effects of these are a bit more uncertain, but one recent study compared several drugs, including a couple of minor tranquillizers, diazepam and phenprobamate, as well as reserpine, a drug that was once used to treat psychotic illness [70]. It was found that, compared with a series of control nights, all three of these drugs actually *increased* the proportion of time spent in dream sleep. Another effect of tranquillizers is that they may alter the *kind* of dreams people have. Patients on these drugs sometimes report that their dreams are more vivid and bizarre. This idea has been tested experimentally by analysing the content of the dreams people report after various drugs [72]. To make sure that most of the dreams were recalled the standard procedure was used of taking a continuous record of each subject's brain waves and eye movements throughout the night. Whenever the record showed signs of paradoxical sleep the subject was woken up immediately and asked to describe the dream he had just had. All the dreams were later analysed for their emotional content. It was found that the drugs used increased the amount of emotion expressed in dreams. The antidepressive drug, imipramine, for example, significantly increased the number of dreams with a hostile or anxious theme. A similar effect was produced by the tranquillizer, prochlorperazine, which also increased the frequency with which people dreamt about sex. Some of the newer drugs, then, either increase the amount of dreaming sleep or make the dreams that do occur more vivid (and by all accounts more interesting!). At the moment we can only guess why these effects occur. One reason, perhaps, is that during the day-time tranquillizers make people less preoccupied with their worries and fantasies, and these find expression after dark.

The world of sleep is a topsy-turvy one, where the rules that apply during waking hours sometimes seem to work backwards; the brain-wave pattern during paradoxical sleep is a good example. We would perhaps be surprised if it were otherwise. Sigmund Freud realized many years ago that sleep and dreaming provide us with an opportunity to act out in utter privacy motives that are sometimes the opposite of those we would confess to in the drawing room. The modern behavioural scientist would put it less appealingly, but the idea is the same. Waking behaviour involves a constant interchange between the nervous system and its environment, a process that is both stimulating and restraining. The brain requires a steady inflow of signals to maintain its vigilance at an adequate level. At the same time its integrated activity depends upon the continuous selection and rejection of signals to be attended to or ignored. In sleep the interchange is between the nervous system and itself, the ticking over of a brain left to its own devices. Under these conditions attention is easily diverted along pathways that are normally inhibited or, as Freud would have said, repressed. Of course, the distinction between sleeping and waking is not as sharp as this and both represent stages along an uninterrupted scale of consciousness. In this chapter we have shown some of the ways in which the individual's behaviour varies as he moves up or down this scale. We have also seen how the changes that occur naturally can be brought under experimental control by the use of psychotropic drugs. Much of the behaviour described has been relatively simple, at any rate about as simple as one can measure without taking a peep inside the head to see what is going on in the brain itself. This is because it is here that one sees most clearly some of the basic features of drug action. The influence of drugs on more elaborate forms of behaviour and conscious experience can then be better understood.

Drugs, Learning and Memory

4

In the previous chapter we saw how psychotropic drugs can influence the individual's level of awareness, so altering his performance on a variety of psychological tasks, especially those demanding a high degree of attentiveness. An important feature of the drug effects described there is that they are relatively short-lived, assuming of course that the drugs are not taken in large doses over a long period of time. Usually once the effect of the drug has worn off performance will return more or less to normal. This is mainly because of the kind of behaviour and laboratory tasks used in studying this particular feature of drug action. Most of the tasks require very little practice to become proficient and, even if they are novel to the subject, he can easily familiarize himself with the procedure before the drug is administered. Choosing simple tasks of this kind is deliberate since here the experimenter is mainly interested in seeing how a change in the subject's physiological arousal will alter the efficiency with which he carries out a particular piece of behaviour. To use tasks on which considerable learning could occur during the experiment itself would only complicate matters unnecessarily, because it might then be difficult to disentangle permanent practice effects from the temporary effects of the drug. As an alternative to using novel, but simple, laboratory procedures the experimenter could equally well choose to study some more complicated but well-ingrained habit, such as driving or walking, where further learning is unlikely to occur after the drug is taken. Here, too, a single dose of most psychotropic drugs will produce effects that are of a temporary, reversible nature – a fortunate outcome for those of occasionally inebriate gait!

Naturally the psychopharmacologist is not only interested in such reversible drug effects as those described so far. Sometimes he may wish to know whether a particular drug has a more permanent influence on behaviour by altering the individual's ability to learn new skills or new responses. For example, he may decide to find out how drugs affect the acquisition of complicated motor skills involving difficult eye-hand coordination. A typical task may consist of learning to keep two randomly moving pointers in alignment or a rod in contact with a rapidly rotating disc. Three matched groups of subjects may be used and, before practising on the task, each will be given a different treatment; say a depressant drug, a stimulant drug, or a placebo. The most likely outcome of the experiment is that subjects given the stimulant will improve more rapidly on the task and reach a higher level of performance than those in the placebo group; while subjects given the depressant will be inferior to both [21].

At the other extreme of complexity the experimenter may be concerned with the effect of drugs on a very simple kind of learning, typically the conditioning of a reflex like the eye-blink response. If an unconditioned stimulus, a puff of air blown at the eye, is associated a number of times with a neutral stimulus, such as a tone, an eye-blink will eventually begin to appear when the tone is presented by itself. The rate at which this takes place can be influenced by psychotropic drugs. Thus, amphetamine will increase and amobarbital will decrease the number of conditioned eye-blinks [27]. Similarly, extinction of the response will be affected by the two drugs. The conditioned eye-blink is normally maintained by giving occasional reinforcement in which the puff of air is also presented, as in the original training procedure. Withdrawal of this reinforcement causes the learned response gradually to disappear, but this extinction will occur more rapidly in subjects given amobarbital than in those given amphetamine.

In studying the effect of drugs on learning, the psychopharmacologist employs research strategies that are similar, at least in principle, to those described in the previous chapter. That is to say, he chooses what he thinks is the best combination of drug and experimental task that will throw into relief a particular aspect of learning or memory. In this way he can begin to isolate different mechanisms involved in the learning process and at the same time begin to understand how drugs differ in their action. In practice, however, compared with the relatively straightforward drug effects discussed in the previous chapter, the influence of drugs on learning and memory is much more difficult to study. This is because drugs do not act in a simple fashion on learning, which is itself a complicated process anyway. It is particularly true of the type of learning that is most relevant to the study of human behaviour and which has been of special interest to psychopharmacologists; namely, the learning of verbal or, to put it more generally, symbolic material. Here, as we shall see, the experimenter may need to exercise considerable ingenuity when designing studies to determine the precise effects of a drug on learning or memory.

We can appreciate some of the problems involved in this area of drug research if we look briefly at what happens during learning. Psychologists have traditionally viewed learning and memory as a continuous process which nevertheless goes through several distinct stages, each stage probably being determined by a different neural mechanism. Three such stages have been recognized, namely those of registration, retention and recall – the three Rs for short. During the initial part of acquisition many of the connexions that could be learned will be rejected and never get beyond the first registration stage. Those that do will pass on to what is now recognized as a two-phase process of retention. The early phase, that of short-term memory, is thought to consist of a relatively brief perseveration or reverberation of the memory trace. During this period, which has been variously estimated as lasting for anything from a few minutes to an hour or so, the memory trace is in an unstable form and can easily be disrupted. However, it gradually becomes consolidated and passes into a more permanent form in the so-called long-term memory store. Retrieval during the recall stage may be either from the short-term or the long-term stores depending on the interval that has elapsed since the original learning. In some cases, in fact, the memory trace may not be permanently stored at all. A good example is the telephone number we need to remember only for a few seconds while we transfer it from the directory to the telephone dial.

Psychotropic drugs can, of course, affect any of the stages of learning just described. What is more important, they may act in a different way at each stage, a given drug perhaps depressing registration but facilitating retention or improving short-term but disrupting long-term memory. The overall result will therefore depend on which phase of learning or memory is mainly affected. Because most drugs have a fairly long time-course of action, their effects will actually tend to spread over two or more stages, depending on when during learning they are administered. How, then, does the psychopharmacologist pinpoint exactly which phase of learning or memory is being influenced by a drug? Some ingenious experiments by Steinberg and Summerfield at London University illustrate one way of going about it.

They were interested in the effects of depressant drugs on the acquisition and recall of verbal material. It is known that people learning such material, or trying to remember it after a short interval, generally perform poorly when under the influence of common sedatives such as alcohol and the barbiturates. However, in previous studies the original learning and later recall had both been tested while the subjects were still affected by the drug. Steinberg and Summerfield argued that depressant drugs may just impair the individual's ability to retrieve information from the memory store and not actually disrupt registration and retention of verbal items. The only way to decide between these two possibilities would be to test for recall of the items *after* the drug effect had worn off. If conventional sedatives were used this would mean waiting at least a day before testing the subjects again, a procedure that would introduce many unwanted complications, such as variations in the extent to which the subjects rehearsed the items during the interval, changes in their motivation, and so on. Steinberg and Summerfield therefore solved the problem by choosing a drug with a very short time-course of action. The drug was nitrous oxide or 'laughing gas' which has the advantage that it does not accumulate in the body but is expired rapidly through the lungs. The subject's level of consciousness can thus be accurately controlled from minute to minute. The gas can be administered, its effects measured, and shortly after it is withdrawn the subject returns more or less to normal. It is therefore an ideal drug for the experiments to be described.

In their first experiment Steinberg and Summerfield had subjects breathe a mixture of nitrous oxide and oxygen during learning and then, soon after withdrawal of the gas, the experimenters tested their subjects' recall of the learned material [63]. The task was one traditionally used in psychological investigations of human memory, namely a list of nonsense syllables. These are meaningless three-letter items, such as BEP, SIJ, KAZ, which are made up so that they have little or no prior association value for the subject. A list of fifteen such syllables was used, the items being exposed through the small window of a rotating memory drum. The subjects were instructed to learn the list by the method of serial anticipation; that is to say, they had to name the next syllable that was about to appear in the memory drum window. Two groups of subjects took part, a gas or experimental group and a control group. To control for the effect of wearing an anaesthetic mask, subjects in the latter group were administered gas-free air throughout the experiment.

In order to check that the two groups were matched for initial ability, all of the subjects breathed air alone for the first four trials of learning, that is for the first four complete presentations of the nonsense syllable list. For the next eleven trials the control group continued to breathe air, while the experimental group was switched to gas conditions. All subjects were then given a rest for two and a half minutes, after which both groups breathed air for a further twenty-five learning trials.

The results of this experiment are shown in Figure 4.1. It can be seen that throughout the period before the rest, when subjects in the experimental group were breathing nitrous oxide, their performance was well below that of control subjects. Is this a permanent effect on learning? The performance curves after the rest suggest that it is. Even when the drug had worn off gas subjects were still inferior, though with further practice under air alone they were finally able to catch up with the control group. The experimenters were therefore able to conclude that nitrous oxide, at least, does not simply impair information retrieval but actually depresses the acquisition of verbal material.

In a second experiment Steinberg and Summerfield again exploited the short time-course of nitrous oxide in order to see how depressant drugs affect the critical phase just after learning has taken place [67]. This involved administering nitrous oxide, not during acquisition itself, but during a short rest interval placed in the middle of a learning session. The idea was to see whether breathing gas would influence the amount of forgetting that occurred over the interval. Their guess was that nitrous oxide

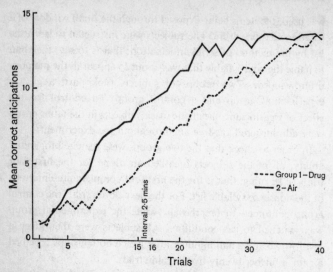

Fig. 4.1. Effect of nitrous oxide on learning nonsense syllables. For the first four trials and the last twenty-five trials – i.e. after the rest – both groups breathed air. During trials 5–15 the drug group breathed nitrous oxide. Note the depressant effect of the drug on learning during this period and persistence of the effect even after the drug group was switched to air.

(Reproduced by permission of H. Steinberg.)

would *reduce* forgetting, this hypothesis being based on the argument that forgetting takes place partly because of inter-ference with the retention process by other neural activity. It is known, for example, that more is remembered if learning is followed by a period of relative quietude or sleep. To see whether nitrous oxide would have a similar effect subjects performing under different sequences of gas and air were given the nonsense syllable learning task described earlier. The learning session was divided into two halves consisting of fifteen trials, followed by a rest for twelve and half minutes and then a continued period of learning for a further twenty-five trials. Three groups of subjects were used. One group, designated air/air, breathed air throughout the first stage of learning and during the subsequent rest. A second, the air/drug group, was changed to nitrous oxide during the rest interval. The third, drug/drug, group breathed nitrous oxide throughout both the initial learning and the interval – except, that is, for four trials on air at the beginning of the experiment. After the rest interval all of the subjects performed under air conditions.

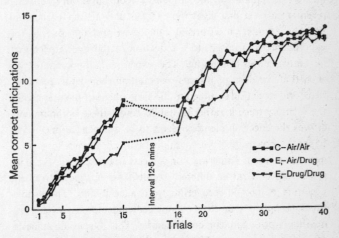

Fig. 4.2. Effect of nitrous oxide on forgetting during nonsense syllable learning. All groups breathed air for the first four trials and for all trials after the rest interval. During trials 5–15, and during the rest, subjects breathed one of three permutations of nitrous oxide or air (see legend). Compare particularly the two upper learning curves, of Groups C and E1, respectively. Note the superior performance of Group E1 after the rest. This was due to forgetting being reduced by subjects breathing nitrous oxide during the interval.

(Reproduced by permission of H. Steinberg.)

Figure 4.2 shows that nitrous oxide had the anticipated effect on forgetting. Comparing the learning curves for the air/air and air/drug groups it can be seen that the performance of subjects who breathed air during the interval had deteriorated by the time they entered the second phase of the experiment. This decline was not evident in those who spent the interval breathing nitrous oxide. As expected from the results of the earlier experiment, subjects who actually learned under the drug performed poorly throughout. However, even they seemed to benefit from continuing to breathe nitrous oxide during the rest interval, since they showed a slight improvement on restarting the task.

Here, then, we find a depressant drug having opposite effects on two aspects of learning, impairing acquisition but improving recent recall. At first sight the effect of nitrous oxide on recall perhaps seems a bit surprising but it was probably due, as the experimenters surmised, to a reduction of the interference that normally causes forgetting. The experimental procedure was such that the dose of nitrous oxide administered was relatively weak and its action confined to the early phase of retention when the memory trace is rather unstable. Under these optimum conditions the effect on memory seems to be a beneficial one. What happens, however, if we administer much larger doses of a depressant drug, rendering our subjects unconscious? There we might expect a rather different result if we can judge from the accounts of people recovering from anaesthetics. They sometimes complain that they cannot remember recent events immediately prior to being anaesthetized. This retrograde amnesia, as it is called, is probably due to the memory trace being disturbed by the rather sudden and profound change in consciousness. Again the very early stages of retention seem to be particularly vulnerable, as the following experiment demonstrates [33].

The purpose of the experiment was to find out whether giving a depressant drug after learning would have a greater effect on subsequent memory than if the drug were administered following a short delay, during which time some consolidation of the memory trace could occur. The subjects were patients about to undergo anaesthesia, induced with the barbiturate, thiopental sodium. Before receiving their anaesthetic the subjects were shown a short picture test, consisting of twenty-four items. Twenty-seven of the patients were then immediately given their injection of the drug. In a further eleven patients, however, the injection was delayed for ten minutes. A day later, memory for the test items was measured by asking the subjects to pick out the original pictures from a larger group containing twenty-four new ones. The results showed that patients given immediate anaesthesia forgot forty-six per cent of the pictures, whereas those given delayed anaesthesia forgot only twenty-one per cent. Thus, memory was less impaired when some consolidation of the traces was allowed to take place by delaying the anaesthetic. Another finding which tended to confirm this conclusion was that the amount of forgetting that occurred depended upon where the pictures were placed in the list. This result is shown in Figure 4.3. It can be seen that, in both groups, pictures early in the list were forgotten less often than those presented later on. In other words, whether a picture was remembered depended on how far away in time it was from the injection. This was presumably because memories of the earlier pictures had a greater chance of being consolidated before the traces were disrupted by the drug.

Of course, we cannot directly compare this experiment with that of nitrous oxide because different drugs and different learning tests were used. However, it seems likely that whether memory is facilitated by depressant drugs depends critically upon the dose administered. In small doses they seem able to protect the memory trace from interference, but in larger amounts this effect is overwhelmed by a disrupting influence on the retention process itself. In this respect anaesthesia is very different from natural sleep, which, as we mentioned briefly earlier, actually increases the amount that is remembered. Why is there this difference? Probably one reason is that anaesthesia involves a rather abrupt loss of consciousness. By comparison the onset of normal sleep is usually a much more gradual affair, beginning with a slow drift through half-wakefulness when organized mental activity is at a low ebb. It is probably this twilight state, occurring at a critical time after learning, that is the important

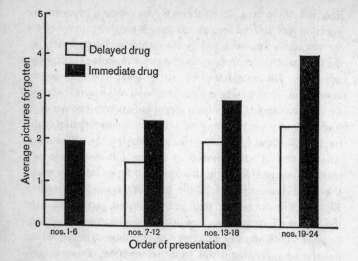

Fig. 4.3. Effect on memory of giving an anaesthetic immediately after learning, compared with delaying administration of the drug for ten minutes. Diagram shows the number of pictures subsequently forgotten under the two conditions, grouped according to their position in the order of presentation. Delaying the anaesthetic reduced the overall amount of forgetting; while in both groups more forgetting occurred the nearer in time the pictures were to the point when the drug was administered.

(From results reported by M. Jarvik. Quoted here by permission of the author.)

factor in determining the influence of sleep on memory consolidation. Hence, too, the facilitating effect of nitrous oxide which, in the light dose used in the experiment described, produces a mental state akin to the early stages of sleep.

The two experiments I have just described have been concerned with drugs administered *after* some learning has taken place. We have seen that careful study of such effects can tell us something about the nature of human memory. Outside the laboratory, however, we do not often encounter situations in which drugs are administered in this way. Or if we do the changes they produce are rarely important. To the patient coming round from an operation it is little more than irritating that he cannot immediately remember the anaesthetist's name. The more usual circumstances under which drugs are taken are those typified by the experiments discussed earlier in this chapter; namely where a drug is likely to influence ongoing learning or some experience that has to be recalled. In this situation stimulant and depressant drugs tend, on the whole, to have opposite effects. As we saw in the case of nitrous oxide, depressant drugs administered during learning will reduce the amount of acquisition that takes place, many of the tranquillizers also having this effect. On the other hand, stimulants such as caffeine and the amphetamines will facilitate performance on learning and conditioning tasks and improve retention of recently memorized verbal material. Of course, these generalizations about the different classes of drug are true only in the broadest sense. Many other factors peculiar to the learner, the learning situation, or both together, may modify the usual effect of a drug. Sometimes the effect may actually be opposite to that generally found. An everyday example is seen in the professional man who comes to the psychiatric outpatient clinic complaining of anxiety affecting the efficiency of his work. Prescription of sedative or tranquillizing drugs will often improve his ability to carry out intellectual tasks that rely on memory. The reasons for this reversal of the usual slowing effect of such drugs have already been touched upon in the previous chapter. There we saw how a very high level of anxiety can disrupt simple forms of behaviour, such as performance on a reaction time task. Complex behaviour is even more sensitive to changes in anxiety level and is even more easily disrupted if anxiety gets very high. Thus, the degree of anxiety that will facilitate a simple response will actually interfere with the learning and recall of, say, a difficult list of nonsense syllables. It is easy to see how, in the very anxious individual, reducing physiological arousal with the right dose of sedative drug will at the same time produce an improvement in intellectual performance. It goes without saying that a stimulant drug given in these circumstances may also have the opposite of its usual facilitating effect on learning and memory.

Even if a drug has its more usual effect on learning, the amount of change that occurs will depend on a number of factors that may operate to diminish or exaggerate its normal chemical action. These may include the nature of the learning task, the conditions under which it is learned, and the conscious effort made by the individual to help along or overcome the drug's effect. For example, a very recent American study showed that the degree to which a given dose of drug affects learning depends very much on what was termed the 'demand load' of the task being learned [20]. The experiment involved giving a graded dose of the sedative, secobarbital, to subjects tested on a large number of learning tasks which varied over a wide range of difficulty. It was found that on tasks demanding great effort from the subject even extremely high doses of secobarbital had no effect, whereas simpler forms of learning were progressively disrupted by increasing amounts of the drug. The results of this study actually illustrate a very general principle in psychopharmacology, namely that the psychological state of an individual, particularly his motivation, may be just as, if not more, important than the chemical action of a drug in determining behaviour. Take the everyday case of the prospective examination candidate putting his faith in God and black coffee in the hope that by the next morning rather less than usual will have escaped his memory store. His belief in the efficacy of caffeine is probably misguided, for whether much is retained or not will depend more on his drive to please the examiners than on any real effect of the drug. In fact, he could probably obtain equally good results (and more sleep!) by just organizing his study properly; for example, by spacing out his learning sessions and following them with a period of rest or relaxation in order to help consolidate the memory traces. Needless to say, investment in a cylinder of 'laughing gas' for this purpose is not recommended!

Unlike the unfortunate examinee or experimental subject most adults, of course, spend only a fraction of their time deliberately learning new habits or acquiring new information. Yet memory forms an integral part of all higher nervous activity. Without it the moment-to-moment retention of experience would not be possible, nor would the recall of more distant events. In this respect the brain mechanisms involved usually work smoothly enough, so smoothly in fact that when the occasional lapse of memory does occur we are surprised or irritated. Common examples are the piece of music we cannot put a title to or the close friend's telephone number that just will not come to mind. Most of the time these lapses are due to an inability to retrieve otherwise well-consolidated items of information from the memory store. Sometimes, however, they may happen because in the first place something disrupted the registration and retention of the events we are trying to recall. A situation of this kind in which drugs are implicated is that giving rise to what is vulgarly known as 'Scotchman's head', a post-party syndrome typically suffered by wayward husbands unable to recall the exact bounds of their hospitality the night before. Can their oblivion be attributed to a genuine effect of alcohol? A recent experiment suggests that at least some of it can [34].

The purpose of the experiment in question was to see how far events that occurred during the consumption of alcohol could be later recalled by the subjects taking part. In order to keep the experimental conditions as natural as possible, the investigation was conducted in a free cocktail-party atmosphere. Students attending a regular weekly get-together were divided into two groups, 'wet' and 'dry'. 'Wet' subjects were allowed as much of their favourite alcoholic beverage as they wished, the barman keeping a note of the kind and amount of liquor each individual consumed. 'Dry' subjects agreed – not surprisingly with some reluctance – to stick to soft drinks for the evening. During the course of the evening the subjects were asked to write stories around sets of pictures taken from the Thematic Apperception

Test, or TAT. These pictures illustrate scenes involving people in vaguely emotional situations which the subject can interpret imaginatively in his own way. Twelve pictures were used, divided into three sets of four. The first set, known as TAT I, was presented before the party began. The other two sets, TAT II and TAT III, were presented, respectively, twenty-five and fifty minutes after the commencement of drinking. The following day subjects in both groups were shown all the pictures again and asked to recall the stories they had written the night before.

The main results of the experiment are shown in Figure 4.4. There it can be seen that, compared with dry subjects, wet subjects forgot a greater proportion of stories elicited under alcohol. The effect was particularly marked in the case of TAT III stories written after almost an hour's drinking. The wet subjects remembered only twenty per cent of what they had written, compared with fifty per cent for dry subjects. These overall effects of alcohol were also revealed in two other findings. One was that, as well as recalling less of their stories, wet subjects also remembered fewer of the actual pictures. Furthermore, within the wet group there was a strong relationship between the amount of alcohol drunk and the amount of material forgotten.

A quite different result was found for stories written *before* drinking began, namely TAT I stories. A glance at Figure 4.4 shows that overall the memory of wet subjects for these stories was actually somewhat *better* than that of dry subjects. This finding was confirmed by the results for individual subjects. It was found that the more a person drank immediately after writing his first set of stories the more he remembered of them the next day. This facilitating effect of alcohol on memory is obviously similar to that described earlier for nitrous oxide and it can probably be explained in the same way. Thus, the alcohol probably prevented other stimuli interfering with consolidation during its critical early stages.

So much for the effect of alcohol on the amount that is recalled. What about the kind of things remembered? This was examined

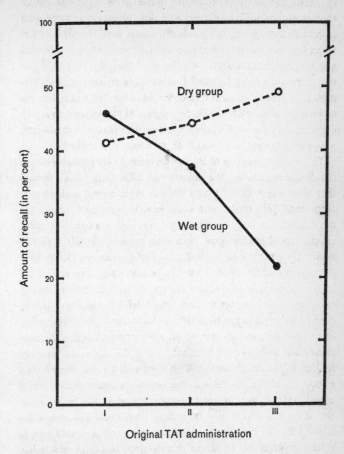

Fig. 4.4. Effect of alcohol on later recall of stories written twenty-four hours earlier. Dry Group drank no alcohol. Wet Group wrote their first stories (Set 1) before beginning to drink and subsequent stories under the influence of increasing amounts of alcohol. Wet subjects later recalled fewer stories written under alcohol but slightly more of those written just before their first drink.

(Reproduced by permission of R. Kalin and the publishers, *Journal of Abnormal and Social Psychology*.)

by classifying the stories according to the themes running through them and then seeing how wet and dry subjects compared with respect to the themes they recalled the next day. The main differences between the groups concerned themes relating to physical sex. Wet subjects forgot these more often than dry subjects when the themes occurred in stories written under alcohol. Furthermore, the greater amount of alcohol an individual drank the less he recalled writing about sex. In the case of stories written *before* drinking, results were again the other way round, wet subjects now remembering more sexual themes than dry subjects.

These selective effects of alcohol on memory are probably due to the drug exaggerating the influence of other, emotional, factors that normally help to decide what is remembered and what is forgotten. Thus, topics with a moderately emotional flavour are more likely to stick in the mind anyway, though like most psychological mechanisms there is an optimum level for this to occur. If events are emotionally *too* highly charged, particularly if they are slightly taboo, they may be selectively forgotten. Now in the experiment just described, the better retention of mildly arousing sexual themes written before drinking began would be even further reinforced by what is at this stage a facilitating effect of alcohol on memory. However, after drinking began the now *depressant* influence of alcohol would be added to another feature of the drug's action. This is its well-known disinhibiting effect, its ability to release the emotions, particularly sexual emotion, from the control of higher centres in the brain. Emotional arousal would now be greater than usual and this, combined with the disruption of memory by alcohol, would lead to selective forgetting of taboo themes once the drug effects had worn off.

Of course, we have no guarantee that the subjects in this experiment had truly failed to retain sexual themes produced under alcohol. They may simply have pushed them out of their mind or, as the psychoanalysts would say, repressed them. Although the idea of repression has been somewhat embroidered by the psychoanalysts there is little reason to doubt that *suppressor* mechanisms, at least, play some part in human memory. After all, most of the material we have available for recall is usually below conscious level. If this were not so mental life would be a kaleidoscopic hell made up of all our past experiences. Technically, repression, as distinct from suppression, is particularly concerned with emotionally charged memories that are pushed further below consciousness than normal so that they are not easily retrieved from the memory store. One of the most dramatic examples of this more powerful form of suppression occurs in the case of complete amnesia following profound emotional shock, as happened in wartime battle-neuroses. The ability of certain drugs to reactivate these 'lost' memories has led to the rather misleading description of them as 'truth drugs'. The term does not, in fact, describe any pharmacologically distinct class of substances. It refers merely to the fact that a variety of drugs, such as the barbiturates, ether, and the stimulant methamphetamine, may have a disinhibiting effect, something like that of alcohol. Their use allows the psychiatrist to reduce conscious control over the emotions and so revive memories which the patient normally finds too painful to recall.

This clinical exploration of memory by drugs takes us a long way from the more sober experimental studies described earlier. It does, however, illustrate the diversity and complexity of drug effects in this area of behaviour. Here drugs are not easily classifiable as stimulant or depressant. The same drug or type of drug may on one occasion facilitate new learning, on another occasion retard it. In yet other circumstances, as we have just seen, it may facilitate in a different way the retrieval of memories that have, if anything, been too well stamped in. At present these various changes can only be isolated by carefully designing experiments in order to bring out or magnify a particular feature of a drug's generally global action on the brain.

Ideally, of course, it would be nice if the research worker could use drugs which were known to have much more precise effects on the different phases of learning and memory. Unfortunately, the action of conventional psychotropic drugs is not as specific as that. Their effects can be likened more to those of a blunderbuss than to those of the marksman's rifle. In the future, however, it may be possible to develop more accurate drug techniques that are applicable to human subjects as we gain further understanding of how the brain processes and stores information. Some progress in this direction has already been made as a result of current research which is trying to identify the physiological and biochemical basis of memory. This research is beginning to give biological reality to such psychological concepts as short- and long-term memory storage. For example, temporary 'holding' of the trace during short-term memory almost certainly involves an important structure in the brain called the hippocampus, located just below the cerebral cortex. It is known, from experiments in which the hippocampus has been damaged or its functions disrupted by drugs, that this area of the brain plays a crucial role in immediate retention.

Transfer of information to the long-term memory store is thought to be associated with physico-chemical changes in the cells of the cortex itself. Any alteration in the state of the neuronal cells is accompanied by a change in the synthesis of their essential biochemical constituents, such as proteins and nucleic acids. It has been suggested that memories are 'coded' and stored in the form of a permanent modification in the molecular structure of these substances, particularly that of ribonucleic acid, or RNA. Support for this theory has come from experiments of several different kinds, some of which involve injecting drugs known to speed up or slow down RNA synthesis, in order to see how learning and retention are affected. Almost all of this work is, of course, carried out on animals, though a somewhat naive hypothesis derived from the RNA theory has already been tested out on human subjects. Several studies have been reported in which elderly patients suffering from memory defects have been fed massive doses of RNA in order to try and improve their mental state. However, these investigations have been so poorly controlled from a scientific point of view that the benefits claimed for this 'treatment' are scarcely justified; especially as it is now known that RNA injected in this way never reaches the brain itself.

Although these RNA experiments on humans have failed, the implication is there: the renovated brain to match the reconditioned body restored to youth with spare-part surgery. That most personal of our possessions has so far eluded the surgeon's knife; or, as a recent correspondent in the *Guardian* put it with rather more feeling, 'we have not yet got brain transplants – thank God!' Mercifully, we probably never will have, at least not as a practical form of treatment. Indeed, the notion is as physiologically crude as it is morally repugnant. But the alternative, an elixir of life for the ageing brain, an instant chemical cure for dementia, is a real possibility, if only in the very distant future. Discovering how to control the intellectual loss associated with old age would certainly represent a major step forward in man's frantic search for the means to immortality. It remains to be seen how easily Nature gives up what may prove to be one of her most important secrets.

A less fanciful but equally controversial development in the field of drugs and learning may occur at the other end of the age-scale. Few of us need reminding of the miseries of our youth when large quantities of factual material had to be committed numbly to memory, a pursuit which, though essential to further educational progress and perhaps somewhat reduced by modern teaching methods, still occupies a disproportionate amount of time, both at school and at university. Given new drugs having quite precise effects on memory and much more knowledge of the learning process itself, it might eventually be possible to reduce considerably the time spent on rote memorization of French verbs and scientific formulae, leaving the educationist greater freedom to develop the more creative talents of his pupils. Such developments in psychopharmacology, combined with more advanced mechanical aids to teaching, may well revolutionize the educational scene of tomorrow.

I leave it to the reader to contemplate the social and ethical problems which both of these advances in drug research will pose for future generations.

A Sober Look at Psychedelics

5

In writing a book of this kind it would be impossible to avoid special mention of the hallucinogenic, psychotomimetic, or psychedelic drugs, as they have been variously called. One of these, LSD-25, I have already discussed briefly and I shall refer to it again from time to time throughout the book. However, the hallucinogens possess peculiar characteristics of their own which set them apart from other drugs and which deserve a chapter to themselves. There are of course other reasons for devoting a whole chapter to one class of drug. No one living in our swinging psychedelic society needs to be reminded of the controversy surrounding LSD and substances like it. Few drugs have stirred up so much intense feeling or sent so many journalists scurrying for their pens; publicity has combined to establish LSD as the drug that things go hippier with. In such a climate of sensationalism it is sometimes difficult to remember that the hallucinogens have made an important contribution to our understanding of human behaviour and experience. The extent of this contribution is itself open to argument, because even professional users of the hallucinogenic drugs have not been entirely innocent of unfounded claims about their scientific value. Early work with mescaline and LSD-25 promised that here at last was the clue to schizophrenia, here was a kind of chemical key that would unlock the secrets of the most puzzling mental illness to afflict mankind. Unfortunately, this hope was not realized. As we shall see later, the kind of psychosis produced by drugs is not identical with schizophrenia – and there are good reasons why one would not expect it to be. In any case, no one now seriously believes that the biochemical effects of a drug like LSD – complicated as they are – can possibly explain the subtle psychological disorders found in schizophrenia. Nevertheless, there are striking similarities between the model psychoses induced by drugs and naturally occurring illnesses that have made the study of hallucinogens worthwhile. A less defensible claim made for LSD, in particular, concerns its place in psychiatric treatment. The drug has been used for this purpose, especially in the United States, in the belief that it makes psychotherapy more effective by helping the patient gain better insight into his 'real' self. At present there is no factual evidence to support this belief and any benefit that may be derived by an individual case is certainly offset by the risks associated with such a potent drug as LSD. The place of the hallucinogens in psychopharmacology, if they now have a place at all, is therefore almost entirely that of research drugs and it is from this point of view that I shall discuss them.

I shall talk mainly about LSD, or, to give it its proper name, lysergic acid diethylamide; though this drug is only one of a number of substances having similar mind-bending properties.*

---

* The internationally agreed name for LSD is 'lysergide' but in the case of this drug I have departed from the convention followed elsewhere in the book and used the more familiar names, either LSD or LSD-25.

Indeed, almost any drug taken in sufficient quantity can under certain circumstances cause mental confusion of a delirious kind – the DTs of the alcoholic are a good example. However, the term 'hallucinogen' properly covers substances which, when given in relatively small doses, produce the feeling of madness or mysticism that has led to the alternative description of them as 'psychotomimetic', or mimickers of psychosis. The connotation 'psychedelic' literally means mind-manifesting and refers to the ability of these drugs to reveal to the individual states of consciousness that he would not usually experience.

The search for something beyond normal experience has preoccupied man for centuries and he has often turned to drugs in order to try and achieve this unity with the unknown. From time immemorial certain plants have been known to induce states of frenzy and ecstasy and these formed an important part of the tribal and religious rites of many ancient cultures. Some such drugs, notably hashish or marihuana derived from Indian hemp, are still consumed in vast quantities in the East. Other more potent hallucinogenic substances occur naturally in the plants of South America. The best known of these is mescaline, a derivative of the peyote cactus of Mexico. Also from Mexico are the psilocybe mushroom, a natural source of the drug psilocybine, and the famous morning glory seeds, traditionally revered for their divine properties by the Indians of South America.

LSD-25 has a different history because it does not occur naturally, though many of its chemical cousins do. Morning glory seeds, for example, are now known to contain the rather less potent hallucinogen, d-lysergic acid amide. The basic constituent is lysergic acid which is closely related to ergotine and ergotamine, two chemicals found in the parasitic fungus ergot. All of these substances are chemically active but not hallucinogenic and it was not until the Swiss chemist Hofmann, in 1938, added diethylamide to lysergic acid that LSD-25 was born. It was another five years before Hofmann accidentally experimented on himself and discovered the drug's remarkable properties. Its effects have subsequently been found to be very similar to those of the naturally occurring hallucinogens, such as mescaline and psilocybine, and few people who have taken all of these drugs can tell the difference between them.

There is one way, however, in which LSD does differ from the other hallucinogens and that is in the infinitesimal amount required to produce its effect. To get some idea of its potency one only has to realize that a teaspoonful of this harmless looking powder would be sufficient to derange mentally the entire population of a city like Oxford. For experimental purposes with human subjects the average dose used is 100 micrograms, or one hundred *millionths* of a gram, a quantity that can scarcely be seen with the naked eye. With smaller quantities subjective changes can still be felt and the threshold dose has been estimated at around twenty micrograms. Physiological changes can be detected at even lower doses, a minute speck weighing seven or eight micrograms producing a measurable increase in the rate of spontaneous GSR activity. This represents an early sign of the excitant effects of LSD.

After oral administration of the normal experimental dose the changes that occur follow a fairly predictable course and can be divided into four stages. Early signs begin to appear during the first thirty minutes and are mainly physical. These include enlargement of the pupil and complaints of nausea, chilliness, or numbness. The height of the reaction occurs between one and five hours and it is then that the true hallucinogenic effects are experienced. This phase is followed by a period of mental impoverishment lasting several hours as the emotional turmoil and more striking perceptual distortions begin to die down. A final stage may then occur, lasting several days, during which time the individual may notice mild after-effects such as slight mental confusion and a feeling of strangeness about the world.

The course of the 'model psychosis' has been analysed in detail by getting subjects to fill in questionnaires at regular intervals after taking LSD. In one study a comparison was made between LSD and an identical placebo [45]. A comprehensive questionnaire was devised covering the more important physical and mental effects of LSD. At various times during the experimental day subjects in both drug and placebo groups were asked to indicate which symptoms they were experiencing. The subjects also completed the questionnaire on the day before the experiment and on the following morning in order to assess the after-effects of LSD. Figure 5.1 shows how the total number of symptoms reported by the LSD subjects changed over the course of

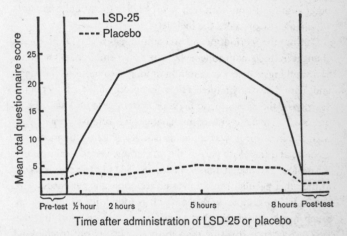

Fig. 5.1. Diagram illustrating the time course of 'symptoms' reported by subjects after taking LSD-25. The curve shown here represents the total number of effects described, but as discussed in the text there is considerable variation in the time course of different effects of the drug.

(Reproduced by permission of H. B. Linton and the publishers, *Archives of General Psychiatry*.)

the day, reaching a peak at about five hours and then gradually decreasing. On average there were only slight after-effects the next day, though one or two subjects reported that they still felt queer.

Figure 5.1 represents the time curve for all of the subjective changes described combined together, but particular kinds of symptom followed a slightly different course. As expected, complaints of bodily discomfort mainly appeared early on, whereas distortions of visual perception reached a peak much later. Within the first half-hour no subjects answered 'yes' to questions like 'Have you been seeing imaginary things?'; but by two hours all of the subjects were admitting that the world around them looked very odd indeed. It is a consistent feature of the LSD state that the bodily discomforts decline in significance as they are superseded by a strange and exciting kaleidoscope of stimuli from other sources. It has been well said of LSD that, unlike alcohol, 'the hangover precedes the inebriety'.

During the period of its maximum effect LSD produces changes in three main spheres of behaviour: emotion, perception, and thinking. Anxiety is common among the emotional changes and, as we saw in Chapter Three, is accompanied by increased activity of the sympathetic nervous system. We also saw there, however, that these autonomic changes are relatively much less than the increase in perceptual sensitivity. Part of the increased anxiety, and therefore part of the autonomic change, that occurs is probably not due to a direct effect of LSD but to apprehension at the other peculiar sensations that the subject experiences as he begins to lose contact with reality. It is found, for example, that much more autonomic change occurs in subjects who find the LSD experience stressing than in those who set out to enjoy it, though both may show an equally marked response to the drug in other ways. The bland, unworried subject is more likely to show other forms of emotional reaction to LSD such as elation or rapid swings between elation and depression.

The perceptual changes that occur are varied and have been well described in the numerous personal accounts of those who have taken the hallucinogens. Briefly, they consist of distortions of size and perspective; increased brightness of colours and intensification of sounds; and a transformation in the appearance of objects, giving rise to illusions or hallucinations. There is a generally heightened awareness of the environment and an uncontrollable flood of sensations and impressions into the nervous system. Another important feature of the loss of perceptual control is the change in the body image, a blurring of the boundaries between the self and its surroundings. Normal perception of the world involves the perception of things in relation to oneself and the appearance of objects remains constant because they can be related to a stable sensation of the boundaries of one's own body. Under hallucinogens the body image is distorted, an effect that has been demonstrated experimentally by getting subjects to estimate the size of parts of their own bodies before and after taking LSD [44]. It was found that under LSD people perceived their heads as being bigger and their arms as being longer than normal. A curious but intriguing experiment!

Turning now to the effects of LSD on thinking, it is not surprising that this highest level of mental activity is disturbed. The individual may feel that thoughts are racing through his head so quickly that they vanish before he has time to string a logical sequence of ideas together. Alternatively, thinking may slow down to the point where ideas seem as though they are stuck to each other. Occasionally, thinking may appear to have stopped completely, producing what is known as a 'thought block' – a fascinating but slightly alarming experience. Under these circumstances it is difficult to perform many intellectual tasks and subjects on LSD invariably show poor memory and concentration and an inability to tackle simple reasoning problems. Part of this disrupting effect is probably due to the individual being distracted by all the other things that are happening to him, but some of it is certainly due to a direct action of the drug on the thinking processes.

One aspect of thinking, however, is popularly believed to be immune to the disrupting effects of LSD, namely creative thinking. Indeed, it has been claimed that creativity is actually heightened during the hallucinogenic experience, an effect that is sometimes put forward by fringe users of LSD as a justification for taking the drug. Artists may claim that they paint better under

LSD or scientists that they gain new insights into problems that were previously insoluble. What evidence is there for this view? Is LSD really capable of releasing submerged creative genius in the most unimaginative of citizens or helping the talented find new dimensions of expression? These questions are particularly difficult to answer because creativity is not an easy thing to measure effectively. By definition it involves the generation of new ideas and has a frustrating habit of disappearing when one tries to devise standardized tests of originality. However, psychologists have made some progress in this direction and it is now possible to measure some of the essential features of creative thinking. Typical tests involve getting the person to think of unusual uses for common everyday objects or asking him to find associations between words that are not normally linked together. Another test which is known to be related to originality is the ability to find a simple geometrical figure when it is hidden in a complex design. A recent experiment studied the effect of LSD on the performance of some of these tests [77]. Subjects were given either LSD or a distilled water placebo and tested twice, once before and once after receiving their respective 'treatments'. Some subjects were slightly more original on the tests after taking LSD, but on the whole there was very little improvement that could be put down to the drug. On one test the LSD subjects did rather worse, in fact. There the subjects were given a set of mosaic tiles and asked to make patterns which were then rated for their aesthetic and creative quality by a group of independent judges. The patterns made while under LSD were rated as generally more disorganized and less original than those made under control conditions. The experimenters concluded that when given to a random group of people, as the subjects of this study were, LSD is unlikely to make them more creative.

It might be argued that tests of the sort used in this experiment could not possibly measure such a complex and highly personal ability as creativeness; and surely creative individuals are not just ordinary people, but a breed apart. Neither of these objections is supported by the facts. Creativity, like other intellectual abilities, is present in everyone to a greater or lesser extent. So-called creative individuals simply possess more of it than most other people. Furthermore, the tests devised to measure original thinking have been found to predict success in occupations that are generally regarded as requiring a high degree of creative ability.

If the reader is not convinced let us consider a quite different study in which both LSD and mescaline were given to a small group of American artists who were considered to be of national importance [4]. The artists were given the opportunity to draw or paint as much as they wished, both before and after taking each of the drugs. After both mescaline and LSD all of the artists experienced the usual feeling of being bombarded by sensory impressions and of being more aware that sounds were louder and colours more vivid. Only one expressed any strong desire to paint and did so with great fervour. An independent panel of fellow artists (presumably not under the influence of the drug!) judged the paintings to be rather more colourful and relaxed in style. The general effect of both drugs, however, was to inhibit the artists and depress their usual painting activities. They reported that painting and drawing were fatiguing and described a disinclination to put brush to canvas or pen to paper. As can be seen from the examples shown in Figure 5.2 the creations they did produce tended to be crude and lacking in detail, or just plain bizarre. An author who also took part in the study experienced a similar feeling of detachment and lack of desire to write. He reported feeling dissatisfied with a play he had written before taking LSD, but felt unable to improve it and totally unconcerned about the human problems it portrayed.

Of course, even this study had certain shortcomings in that the individuals taking LSD were doing so under conditions that were inevitably somewhat mentally restricting. However much the experimenters tried to make the atmosphere as free and relaxed as possible, their subjects were nevertheless being asked to create

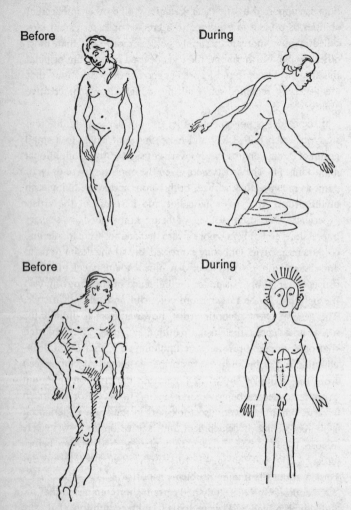

Fig. 5.2. Examples of drawings done by the same professional artist before taking LSD and while under its influence.

(Reproduced by permission of H. Goodell and co-authors and the publishers, *Journal of Nervous and Mental Disease*.)

at will, which most people suppose is a difficult thing to do. Perhaps we should therefore let a creative artist speak for himself on the topic, in this case one of the world's most talented film directors, Federico Fellini. In an interview for the contemporary arts magazine, *Envoy*, Fellini was asked whether he thought that the use of hallucinatory drugs can enrich the creative process. In his reply he commented [22]:

No hallucinatory drug can add to the imagination of someone who is completely lacking in imagination. No drug can make imagination. It would be too easy if all you had to do was to take LSD to become a visionary or a prophet. The experience itself can be interesting, captivating or highly dangerous, but I do not believe in its use for creative purposes.

There is no evidence, then, that hallucinogens provide a short-cut to creative talent; while there is scarcely any more evidence that they can benefit those people who are already highly creative. This is not to say that in any given individual such drugs cannot break down inhibitions, leading to freer expression of ideas and feelings. But that effect is common to many drugs, including alcohol, and is probably not specific to the hallucinogens. The latter are, in fact, more likely to disorganize creative thinking because of their disrupting influence on what is a highly integrative mental process.

There is, of course, a slightly different way in which drugs like LSD could perhaps help the creative individual. The hallucinogenic state could conceivably give him new perceptions or new insights which he might recall when the immediate effects of the drug itself have worn off. These might be incorporated in a work of art subsequently created in a drug-free state. Whether the painting or other artistic effort that resulted were considered unusually creative would then have to be judged by the same standards as those applied to any other work of art affected by life experience. I suspect that in most cases their quality would be somewhat akin to the ideas that come into our heads just as we drop off to sleep - brilliantly conceived at the time, but stupidly banal when viewed in the grey light of morning. However, it is worth mentioning one, particularly laudable, example of how insights gained through taking LSD can be put to creative ends. It concerns the application of the drug to architecture. Over ten years ago a Canadian architect, Kiyoshi Izumi, asked himself how one should build a hospital specifically suited to the needs of the mentally ill. He decided that one way to find out was to take LSD. This, he felt, would tell him something of how the schizophrenic perceives the world and how deficiencies in the mentally ill person could be compensated for in building design. Izumi's experiences of LSD were characterized by the now familiar perceptual distortions, described in the following way by Jackson House who covered the story for the *Canadian Weekly* [32]:

In his pseudo-schizophrenic state, Izumi believed time was standing still although he saw the hands of clocks moving. Corridors seemed to go on and on, into eternity. He remembers that 'noises reverberated through the building and were extra loud. People's faces kept changing, sometimes blending and disappearing into the background. There was too much contrast in the checker-board pattern on the floor. I felt I was walking up the squares on a pedestal, raising my feet higher than I had to. The floor tended to rise and go down. The cracks between the planks looked like canyons, very deep and cavernous. I saw a patterned covering on a chesterfield and the patterns moved in and out.'

From his analysis of the LSD state Izumi developed new concepts of design for building mental hospitals which have since been put into practice in various parts of Canada and the United States. One new hospital finished in 1963 in Yorkton, Saskatchewan and incorporating many of Izumi's revolutionary ideas, is described by Jackson House in the following way:

There is hardly a sound as the inmate walks from cottage to cottage . . . Hidden sounds – Izumi found noises too loud, their sources hard to identify – like fans, furnace motors, echoing surfaces, switches, have been eliminated. The patient can enter the dayroom unobtrusively, from the side, and join a group if he wishes without being stared at. The whole hospital is decorated in muted colours . . . which contribute to the general air of tranquillity. There are no patterns in drapes, walls, upholstery – patterns that could turn into hostile images . . . Windows project outwards to allow him 'visual escape' into the outdoors unobstructed by other walls or buildings. Floors are smoothly tiled – there are no cracks between planks that could turn into Izumi's 'canyons, very deep and cavernous'. There are no polished tiles, multiple mirrors or other shiny surfaces where an inmate might see his own image, frightening, distorted.

This unusual and humanitarian use of LSD in creative art contrasts markedly with the somewhat egocentric introspection which seems to motivate much of the search for creative insight through hallucinogenic drugs. It also illustrates one of the ways in which hallucinogens can help us understand some of the problems faced by the schizophrenic patient, a point I will take up in more detail later. First, however, let us look at some more general features of the LSD state as it occurs in the normal individual.

The general effects of the hallucinogens described so far can be modified on any particular occasion by a number of social and psychological factors; though one thing one would not expect is a placebo response to the drug. LSD is so powerful and its effects so unmistakable that an imagined reaction to it is scarcely credible. However, such responses to LSD are by no means unknown and this is how one individual, given a harmless placebo, described his LSD 'psychosis' [51]:

A lot of strange shapes and brilliant colour, after-images, as if I looked through pebble finished glass, particularly this morning. Especially this morning colours were more brilliant than I have ever experienced. Voices were at times somewhat in the distance along with a feeling of not being in a real situation, a dream kind of state, time is distorted, goes rather slowly, an hour is only 10 or 15 minutes when I look at my watch.

A perfect description of the LSD state! Interestingly enough, when this subject was told what he had been given and then a week later given a normal dose of LSD he reported that the drug had no effect at all. Perhaps distilled water, dispensed with appropriate ceremony, is, after all, the answer to man's search for the occult!

Apart from the individual's expectations about what will happen to him, the surroundings in which the hallucinogens are taken will also modify their effect. In a barrenly furnished laboratory the perceptual experiences may be dull and disappointing because there will be little variety in the stimuli that can be distorted. An extreme example occurs under conditions of sensory deprivation where the input of stimuli is drastically reduced. These conditions are produced experimentally by putting subjects in a sound-proofed room cut off from human contact and getting them to wear goggles on their eyes and cuffs on their arms, all of which combine to isolate the brain from a good deal of the information that is necessary for its proper functioning. The normal effects of sensory deprivation are very like those of LSD. The individual loses track of time, shows poor concentration and mental control, and experiences visual illusions of various kinds. The similarity between the two conditions is interesting because it means that they both probably affect the brain in the same way, causing a breakdown in its processing and integrating mechanisms. When the two are added together and subjects undergoing sensory deprivation are given LSD, many show little reaction to the drug. It is as though when the input to the brain is already severely limited not much scope is left for the hallucinogens to exert their usual effect. However, not everyone reacts like this to the combination of LSD and sensory deprivation. Some people may show a more marked response to the drug than usual. This is probably because some individuals are more dependent on stimulation from their environment than others. They will find sensory deprivation unpleasant anyway and the drug will simply exaggerate its already uncomfortable effects.

In addition to the physical environment, the social surroundings will influence the reaction to LSD and other hallucinogens. This, of course, is true of any drug, the most familiar example being alcohol, which is by no means as pleasant for the solitary drinker as for the party-goer. In the case of the hallucinogens the effect is more complicated because they have a more widespread influence on behaviour anyway. Just as the individual's perception of objects is enhanced by LSD, so too is his sensitivity to the people around him. This is seen even in the controlled conditions of the laboratory. In our own studies of LSD, which have been mainly concerned with the physiological effects of the drug, subjects have responded in various ways to our sober, white-coated appearance. A few have reacted with suspicion, feeling that they were guinea pigs in some diabolical experiment. Others have regarded us with barely veiled amusement at the stupidity of our interest in their pulse rates when so many much more interesting things were happening to them! As one would expect, when several people take hallucinogens together the drug effects are modified considerably. The dangers and delights of the LSD party stem from the fact that the drug's action adds to and exaggerates the prevailing mood of the group and the existing attitudes of its members towards each other. One American study which looked at the effects of giving LSD to people in small groups found that there was a marked reduction in anxiety feelings, but an increase in suspiciousness about others in the group [61]. Compared with individuals who took the drug alone, 'group' subjects were more active and elated, and less introspective about their own symptoms. They also reported fewer perceptual distortions, though the overall severity of the model psychosis was not altered. The experience was generally less distressing and the authors concluded that it was reassuring for subjects to have a fellow traveller into the unknown; or, as they put it, 'To be different alone is to be crazy or eccentric, but to be different together is merely to be exclusive.'

The most powerful factor influencing the reaction to hallucinogens is the personality of the individual taking them. Unfortunately, having said this it is difficult to say anything much more precise. If it were possible then we should know very much more than we do at present both about personality and about the action of LSD. Observing other people under LSD the feeling is strongly one of 'I told you so'. There is a conviction that had one known more about the hidden subtleties of their personalities it would have been possible to predict more accurately beforehand how they would react to LSD. In a crude way this can be done already, the general effect of LSD being to exaggerate existing personality traits. Thus, the calmly introverted become preoccupied with their own thoughts, the cheerful extravert quips and puns his way through an elated few hours, and the tense describe distressing bodily symptoms of anxiety. Some of these observations are supported by experimental evidence that people of rather rigid and inflexible personality, who also score highly on questionnaires of depression and neurotic introversion, tend to react more severely to and enjoy the hallucinogenic experience less than those of more relaxed and free and easy disposition. Much has been written, especially by psychoanalytic authors, about the use of LSD to explore the underlying dynamics of the personality. It is this use of the drug that is mainly responsible for unfounded claims about its effectiveness in psychiatric treatment and its present notorious status as a chemical aid to instant insight. My feeling is that most of what has emerged could have been discovered in other ways with considerably less trouble to society.

There is another more restricted sense in which it has been argued that LSD has made a serious contribution to our knowledge of personality. This concerns the similarity between the hallucinogenic experience and schizophrenia, the so-called 'psychotomimetic' quality of the LSD state. In the present climate of opinion about hallucinogens it is reasonable to ask whether the results of over twenty years' research in this area justify the continued study of these controversial drugs. How similar to schizophrenia are the effects produced by LSD? If the two states are not identical, are they sufficiently similar to tell us anything at all about natural mental illness? The answers to these questions concern both layman and scientist. Neither is immune to the group of illnesses that LSD is supposed to mimic and which afflict nearly one per cent of the population. Yet both have reached a point of crisis where the term 'psychedelic' provokes a reaction almost as irrational as that produced by the hallucinogens themselves. Some scientists are wary of pursuing research on LSD as long as the ethics of its use are at issue. At the same time they are loath to abandon it completely if there is any likelihood at all that it will bring the solution to schizophrenia a little nearer. The dilemma is an ironic one because, just as society 'discovered' LSD, so the drug's interest to psychopharmacology began to wane as it met the fate of many breakthroughs in science and entered a phase where cautious optimism or even pessimism replaced intense enthusiasm for its value as a tool in psychiatric research. This is a particularly appropriate time to consider whether the hallucinogens still have a place in the study of schizophrenia.

That LSD produces psychotic behaviour is beyond dispute. So, however, do many other insults to the brain, including direct injury, infection, or large doses of drugs not classified as hallucinogens, such as amphetamine. All of these have slightly different effects from each other and from schizophrenia. The most that can be said of the hallucinogens is that they come closest of all to imitating the symptoms of schizophrenia. As we shall see later, although particular symptoms that occur under LSD may be typically schizophrenic, it is rare in any given individual for the total model psychosis to duplicate the natural illness. Thus, the LSD subject may show signs of catatonia, that is to say he may become withdrawn and physically immobile; but he is unlikely to show all of the symptoms that would lead a psychiatrist to diagnose him as suffering, even temporarily, from the catatonic form of schizophrenia.

There are several reasons why model and natural psychoses are not exactly the same. One simple reason is that there are a few symptoms that occur in schizophrenia which are not very common in the normal person who takes LSD. A notable example is the auditory hallucination. 'Hearing voices' is often found in schizophrenia, but is rarely experienced in the LSD state, where most of the perceptual distortions are visual. This may be an important difference because it has been suggested that in some forms of schizophrenia there may be a disturbance in areas of the brain that store and process auditory information. Studies of schizophrenic patients have shown, for example, that their performance is especially impaired when they are asked to carry out psychological tasks under auditory distraction. Such patients also seem to have difficulty in coding auditory information of a meaningful kind, a fact which probably partly accounts for the schizophrenic's inability to communicate with other people and his frequent complaint that he cannot follow the track of normal conversation. Since LSD does not often produce such marked effects in auditory perception, this alone limits what we can learn from it about the abnormalities of brain function responsible for schizophrenia.

Another reason for the dissimilarity of the model and natural psychoses arises from the conditions under which they occur. In the one case an otherwise normal individual takes a drug, the effects of which last for a few hours. During this time he is usually fully aware that he is under the influence of a drug and can often, if necessary, shrug off its effects and return more or less to his normal self. In other words, there is not the complete disintegration of personality that is present in schizophrenia. The schizophrenic patient, on the other hand, is someone in whom difficulties in communication, thinking, and emotional expression have become built into his personality through a gradual deterioration of mental life which may have persisted over many years and indeed may never have been normal. Where the schizophrenic reaction has a very sudden onset, as sometimes happens, the similarity with model psychosis will be greater. However, even here it will not be perfect because of differences in the way in which the person deals with the experience. One will occur out of the blue in a vulnerable individual who can muster few reserves of personality to cope with all the frightening things that are happening to him. The other will occur in a normal individual volunteering to undergo an experience which, however alarming, he is pretty sure will end sooner or later. The reader can perhaps get some idea of the difference between the two situations if he imagines what it might be like if he were given LSD without being aware of it and its effects were maintained over a long period of time.

Despite the fact that drug-induced and natural psychosis differ fundamentally in quality, the two conditions still show some remarkable similarities. This can be illustrated by comparing individual symptoms of the LSD state with those described by schizophrenic patients in the early stages of their illnesses. Dr James Chapman in Dundee has made a careful and invaluable study of what the schizophrenic experiences as he becomes psychotic. As we shall see in a moment, some of the accounts given by patients he has interviewed bear a striking resemblance to those reported by normal people after taking hallucinogens [11]. Indeed, they are so similar that few experts in the field, reading them out of context, could distinguish between them. The following, for example, is an extract from one patient's description of how his visual perception became distorted as he became ill:

I was sitting listening to another person and suddenly the other person became smaller and then larger and then he seemed to get smaller again. He did not become a complete miniature. Then today with another person, I felt he was getting taller and taller. There is a brightness and clarity of outline of things around me. Last week I was with a girl and then suddenly she seemed to get bigger and bigger, like a monster coming nearer and nearer. The situation becomes threatening and I shrink back and back.

Another patient described his experience in this way:

I see things flat ... There's no depth, but if I take time to look at things I can pick out the pieces like a jigsaw puzzle, then I know what the wall is made of. Moving is like a motion picture. If you move, the picture in front of you changes.

Both of these accounts could typically have been given by LSD subjects, as could the following patient's description of how thinking was a difficult and laborious process:

I can't shut things out of my mind and everything closes in on me. It stops me thinking and then the mind goes a blank and everything gets switched off. I can't pick things up to memorize because I am absorbing everything around me and take in too much so that I can't retain anything for any length of time – only a few seconds.

The theme running through many of these descriptions, as through accounts of the LSD state, is the feeling of having a constantly changing pattern of stimuli rushing in on the individual; or, as one of Dr Chapman's patients put it, 'Nothing settles in my mind – not even for a second. It just comes in and then it's out. My mind goes away – too many things come into my head at once and I lose control.'

This inability to control attention is probably one of the most significant points of similarity between the effects of LSD and schizophrenia. We can begin to see why this is so if we recall some of the ideas discussed in Chapter Three. There we saw (page 67) how normal attention requires a constant selection and rejection of stimuli, attention narrowing and broadening as the individual becomes more or less aroused. Now, one odd effect of LSD is that attention gets very broad, so that the individual takes in much more information from the environment than he should. This is normally associated with a low level of arousal, as might be induced, for example by a sedative drug. Yet LSD is generally *stimulant* and therefore arousing in its effects and one would have expected attention to get narrower rather than broader. The fact that the opposite happens suggests that LSD in some way disturbs the fine balance that exists between the mechanisms in the brain that control arousal and those controlling attention. As we shall see later in the book (Chapter Seven, page 180), a similar brain disturbance may occur in some forms of schizophrenia, for here too the patient is often anxiously aroused but, like the LSD subject, quite unable to ignore irrelevant stimuli.

Some research workers feel that this disorder of attention is a basic characteristic of schizophrenia that can explain many of the other symptoms of the condition. If they are right, then drugs like LSD could still prove invaluable in bringing important features of the natural illness under experimental control. So far, perhaps understandably, most of the work done on LSD in humans has been concerned with its more exotic subjective effects – and even the pure scientist has to admit that these are the most interesting. Unfortunately, there is a limit to what these effects can tell us objectively about schizophrenia and if, as I believe, the hallucinogens still have an important contribution to make to the study of mental illness, the behavioural scientist will have to return to his laboratory and continue from there the long painful process of scientific discovery. However, before doing so he could with advantage – and under careful supervision – take LSD once in order to get some insight into the human problem he is trying to solve. A personal anecdote will illustrate the value of this experience to anyone, in fact, whether research worker or therapist, who is professionally involved with the schizophrenic patient.

Some years ago, as part of a research project on schizophrenia, I was interested in a visual illusion called the Archimedes spiral after-effect. The illusion is measured by getting the subject to keep his eyes fixed on a rotating disc which consists of a thick black spiral drawn on a white background. While it is rotating the spiral normally appears to be moving outwards from its centre, giving the disc a slightly three-dimensional quality. On one occasion I was giving this test routinely to a young schizophrenic patient when quite suddenly he leapt forward out of his chair and, with a look of terror in his eyes, he struck the appara-

tus to the ground. He explained afterwards that he was frightened
that he would become enveloped by the spiral as it emerged from
the disc. My reaction was one of sympathy without real understanding of what the patient had told me. Several years later, long
after I had forgotten this patient, I took LSD in connexion with
some subsequent research on hallucinogenic drugs. At the point
where I was beginning to get the usual visual distortions a colleague decided he would like to measure my spiral after-effect.
While I was staring at the disc the rotating spiral took on an
alarming, almost menacing appearance, accompanied by unpleasant bodily sensations due to synaethesia – a common effect
of LSD in which stimulation of one sense modality crosses over
and produces impressions in another modality. Memory of this
experience afterwards reminded me of my patient who had tried
so inadequately to explain his behaviour to me. It was not until
then that I really understood what he was trying to tell me.
Indeed, my day on LSD gave me for the first time some appre-
ciation of what the world can look like through the eyes of the
schizophrenic patient. The experience as a whole was a reasonably
pleasant one, but I was impressed by how different it might have
been had it all happened as part of a real schizophrenic illness.

Everyone who has had close contact with schizophrenia knows
of the impenetrable barrier that exists between himself and the
patient. This 'glass wall', as it has been called, makes it difficult
for others to understand the bizarre thoughts and feelings the
schizophrenic is barely able to communicate. The patient may
do inexplicable things, as mine did, prompted by his mispercep-
tion of the world around him. Even the most sympathetic
observer may react with anger or bewilderment. Those who have
taken LSD with the serious intent of gaining more insight into
schizophrenia have also, I believe, achieved a greater tolerance
of this terrible condition. If the hallucinogens make no further
contribution to our knowledge of human behaviour, they will in
this entirely human way have justified an existence that society
has sometimes had occasion to regret.

Why Drug Effects Vary 6

Some time ago a friend of mine was conducting an experiment on the effects of a common psychotropic drug on reaction time. At the end of the experiment, just as the subjects were leaving the laboratory, one of his colleagues happened to pass by. Noticing that one of the subjects looked extremely drowsy he later inquired casually how the experiment had gone and which sedative or tranquillizer was being used. He received the reply, 'That was no sedative; that was amphetamine.'

Paradoxical drug responses of this kind illustrate the difficulty of rigidly classifying psychotropic drugs as depressant, stimulant, tranquillizing and so on. For practical purposes it may be useful to do so, because it provides the psychopharmacologist with a shorthand description of the effects typically produced by different drugs. Whether a drug has its usual effect on a particular occasion will, however, depend on a number of factors which modify its normal action. Often the response to a drug will be greater or smaller than expected. Sometimes it may even be entirely opposite to that predicted, as in the case of the subject I have just described. The reason for this variability is easily understood if one realizes that a drug is just like any other stimulus applied to the organism, its purely pharmacological action interacting with the many other influences that are affecting behaviour at the same time. We have already seen how powerful these non-pharmacological influences can be in the case of the placebo response. In this chapter we shall see how chemically active drugs do not always behave as they should and why their effects vary considerably from one individual or one situation to the next.

Although we shall be concerned here mainly with non-pharmacological factors it should be remembered that the drug itself can also give rise to a good deal of variability. The dose administered will clearly play an important role, though the effects produced may not always be a simple function of dosage. Some depressant drugs, for example, may have excitant properties at low doses, or at critical doses that are different for different individuals. The correct average dose to produce a predominantly depressant effect in a group of subjects therefore has to be chosen with care. Another pharmacological factor of some importance is the manner in which the drug is given, that is whether it is administered orally or by injection. Drugs given by injection will reach their peak effect very quickly and, dose for dose, induce more profound and immediate changes in behaviour. By comparison, those taken by mouth will be absorbed much more slowly, their effects accumulating gradually over a period of time.

In most drug experiments, of course, the dose and route of administration is standardized and the variation in response observed is mainly due to other factors. These non-pharmacological influences can be divided into two types. First, there are those that arise from the situation in which the drug is given, including any expectations induced in the subject about the possible effects of the drug; and secondly, there are those that are due to the individual characteristics of the experimental subjects, such as undue sensitivity and either temporary or permanent resistance to the drug's action.

The potency of psychological influences on drug response has been demonstrated in a number of experiments designed in such a way that the normal effect of a drug is deliberately distorted by giving misleading information to the experimental subjects. Thus a group of subjects may be given a stimulant drug, such as amphetamine, and, with a suitably persuasive spiel, prepared to expect the effects normally produced by depressant drugs. The subjective and objective physiological changes that occur will be in the 'depressant' direction, reports of tiredness and slowness being much commoner than in subjects who are told the truth about the drug they have taken. If no instructions are given about the effects anticipated, then the pharmacological action of even a relatively large dose of a drug may disappear. This was recently demonstrated in a study carried out by Dr Frankenhaeuser and her colleagues in Stockholm [26]. They studied the reactions of subjects under three experimental conditions. Under one condition the subjects were given a placebo and told it would have the typical sleep-producing effects of a depressant drug. Under the other two conditions they were given 200 mg. – a fairly high dose – of pentobarbital, but in one case they were told to expect the normal depressant effects and in the other that the drug might or might not have any effect at all. Various measurements were taken, including reaction time and ratings of subjective feelings under the three treatments. It was found that, despite the dose administered, the drug only had a consistently significant effect when it was combined with the appropriate suggestions beforehand. When given with neutral instructions its action was rather weak, the placebo by comparison being somewhat *more* effective in producing feelings of sleepiness.

In some situations, even though the subject may know the kind of drug he has taken, he may be motivated in such a way or to such a degree that he is able to overcome its effects. No doubt many a merry reader will have experienced the utter sobriety that comes over one when a sudden emergency arises requiring rapid action; as, for example, when a party guest is taken ill. On such occasions the subjective experience may actually be one of remarkable clear-headedness during the period of crisis, as though the alcohol consumed previously had actually speeded up mental processes more than usual. Is this possible? Certainly it has been shown in experimental situations that, if the incentive to perform is strong enough, then the typical slowing effects of depressant drugs may actually be reversed. This was demonstrated in a study carried out in the United States on the effect of pentobarbital on reaction time under different incentive conditions [31]. The subjects were a group of former morphine addicts who, as a strong incentive, were offered a shot of morphine immediately after carrying out the experimental task. With this to motivate them the subjects given pentobarbital actually performed faster than usual, the drug apparently acting on this occasion as a stimulant. On the other hand, when only a weak incentive was offered – a morphine injection at some later date – the drug had its more usual depressant effect of slowing down reaction time.

Deliberately manipulating the individual subject's motives or expectations is one way, then, in which drug effects can be enhanced, diminished, or reversed. Other important influences will arise from the natural setting in which the drug is taken. If several people in a group take the same drug, then each person's response to it will act as a stimulus to other members of the group. This interaction may bring out features of the drug's action that are not apparent in people taking the drug alone. It is well-known that the solitary drinker rarely experiences the party spirit. He just gets more and more morose. The influence of social interaction on drug response is by no means confined to human groups, but can also be demonstrated in animal colonies. Thus, a very small dose of amphetamine given to a colony of mice may cause a significant increase in group activity, even though the same dose may have no detectable effect on the behaviour of an individual animal tested in isolation. Comparable effects have also been produced by administering depressant drugs. A dose of barbiturate which will normally heavily sedate a single animal may actually make a colony of mice much more active.

Group-interaction effects on human drug response have been studied in some ingenious experiments which have tried to isolate the separate influence of pharmacological and social factors. In some of these experiments small groups of, say, four subjects are used. On some occasions all of the group members will be given the same drug, either a stimulant or a depressant. Alternatively, drugs having opposing pharmacological effects will be given to different people in the same group, half of them being given a stimulant and the other half a depressant drug. As one might expect, when everyone in the group takes the same drug, its effects on behaviour tend to be exaggerated by the additional stimulus of social interchange within the group. Either the drug's normal action is magnified or its effects reversed. However, if drugs of opposite type are used in the same group of people they may cancel each other out. Thus, a person receiving a stimulant, for example, may not experience its usual effects when he is required to interact with someone receiving a depressant drug. This dilution of drug action has been named, rather appropriately, the 'wash-out' effect.

A particularly neat example of the kind of experiment just described is one carried out by Dr Starkweather at the University of California [62]. He was interested in the effect of giving different drug combinations to people working in pairs on a simple psychological task. The task was one called the trail-marking test which consists of numbers and letters scattered randomly over a page. The subject was required to join the numbers and letters in alternating sequence, joining 1 to A, A to 2, 2 to B, and so on. His score was the time taken to complete the test. The basic design of the experiment involved testing each subject individually both before and after an interval during which he cooperated with another subject on a modified version of the trail-marking test. In this modified form the test was adapted so that two people could do it together, each member of the pair being given half the information necessary to complete the task. Each was able to communicate his 'moves' to his opposite number by a system of coordinates which allowed him to indicate the direction and length of the lines drawn to connect particular letters and numbers. This schedule of individual and cooperative testing was repeated at weekly intervals for seven weeks. For three of the sessions all of the subjects were given placebos. For the remaining four they received either phenobarbital or amphetamine. On the drug days during cooperative testing the subjects were paired off in one of three ways. Sometimes both members of a pair were on the depressant, sometimes both on the stimulant, and sometimes one person was on the stimulant and his partner on the depressant. The effect of these different drug combinations was measured by seeing how subsequent performance on the individual version of the trail-marking test compared with that before the interaction experience.

Before carrying out this experiment Dr Starkweather made certain predictions about its outcome. These are shown in Figure 6.1. A fairly straightforward prediction could be made about the drug effects before the subjects were allowed to interact with each other. As seen in the left half of the diagram, it was simply predicted that performance would be worse, that is the task would take longer to complete, on phenobarbital than it would on amphetamine. It was anticipated that, after interaction, performance would change in the directions shown on the right side of Figure 6.1. Where both members of a pair had been on the same drug it was expected that the normal drug effect would be exaggerated, sedated subjects becoming even slower and stimulated subjects becoming faster. When partners had been on opposite drugs it was thought that a 'wash-out' effect would occur, performance afterwards changing to some intermediate level. The actual results are shown in Figure 6.2. Performance before interaction was as predicted, phenobarbital subjects taking

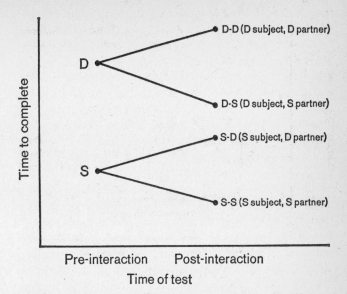

Fig. 6.1. Diagram showing the predictions that were made before an experiment on the effects of interaction between subjects on either a depressant (D) or a stimulant (S) drug. Before interaction D subjects were expected to be slower than S subjects. It was thought that these differences would be exaggerated after subjects had interacted with someone on the same drug. In subjects on opposite drugs performance scores were expected to come together, producing a 'wash-out' effect (see text). Figure 6.2 shows the actual results of the experiment.

(Reproduced by permission of J. A. Starkweather.)

significantly longer to complete the task than amphetamine subjects. After interaction, however, performance changed in a quite unexpected manner. As can be seen in Figure 6.2, pairing off two subjects who were on the same drug actually caused the normal drug effect to be reversed. This was true of both the stimulant and the depressant drug. Thus, stimulated subjects, who showed fast performance on the first testing, were slowed to the level of depressed subjects after working with someone who was also on the stimulant. Similarly, subjects on the depressant were not, as

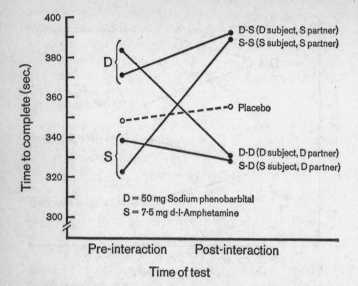

Fig. 6.2. Results of an experiment on the effects of interaction between subjects on either a depressant (D) or a stimulant (S) drug. Differences in the performance of D and S subjects before interaction were as expected (cf. Figure 6.1). After interaction these differences were reversed in pairs on the same drug (D-D and S-S), subjects on the depressant now being quicker than those on the stimulant. Interaction between subjects on different drugs (D-S and S-D) produced the opposite of a 'wash-out' effect.

(Reproduced by permission of J. A. Starkweather.)

anticipated, slowed down further by working with a depressant partner. On the contrary they were speeded up to the stimulant level. The effect of pairing off people who were on different drugs was also rather unexpected. On this occasion a 'wash-out' effect did not occur. Instead, subjects on the depressant who worked with a stimulated partner were slowed down and those on the stimulant who worked with a depressed partner were speeded up. In all cases, then, the differences in performance after interaction were related, not to the drug the subject himself had taken, but to the drug his partner had taken. A partner who took amphetamine consistently slowed down the person he worked with, while a partner on phenobarbital had the effect of speeding up his opposite number. This was true whatever drug the subject himself took and even though before interaction he had shown a typical drug response. This experiment illustrates very well how, in some situations, one's own response to a drug may depend, not so much on its direct pharmacological action, as on the perception of other people's behaviour with whom one is interacting. Or, as Dr Starkweather rather whimsically comments, if we look at it the other way round, perhaps it is the doctor who should take the drugs in order to influence his patients!

Let us turn now to the other important source of variability in drug response, namely the variation that arises from within the individual himself. That people differ widely in their sensitivity to drugs will be obvious to anyone who has relieved the monotony of a cocktail party by observing the reactions of his fellow guests. Some of this variation can be put down to factors of a temporary nature, since even the same person will react differently to the same drug given on different occasions. For example, the nearness and size of his last meal will help to determine how rapidly the drug is absorbed into the blood-stream and hence allowed to reach the brain. The presence of another drug in the body may also be important, one drug often intensifying the effects of another; as in the dangerous combination of barbiturates and alcohol. Another important variable is transient fatigue, which may make the person temporarily more sensitive to a drug than he would otherwise be. A less obvious factor is the individual's mood which will act as a touchstone for the social influences on drug response already described.

Apart from these random fluctuations within the same person, differences between people occur because of a variety of relatively permanent individual characteristics, many of which are purely physical. Weight, for instance, may be important because it is related to the volume of circulating blood, which helps to determine the concentration of drug reaching the brain at any one time. It is for this reason that for clinical purposes weight, or some index taking account of weight, is used as a rough guide to the dose of drug to be administered. For the same reason in experimental studies, instead of giving all subjects the same amount of drug, the dosage is often corrected so that each person receives a quantity proportional to his body weight. Another closely related physical characteristic is the body type, whether the person is fat or thin. Some drugs have a proclivity for fat, attaching themselves, as it were, to fatty tissue in the body and being released gradually from it over a period of time. In a very plump person, therefore, the time-course over which such drugs act will be altered compared with someone of more modest build. Both weight and body type will, of course, be related to age and sex, so that each of these will also indirectly affect the drug response. Physical health may be a further source of individual variability, someone with brain damage, for example, being particularly sensitive to psychotropic drugs. Another factor of some importance is the degree to which the person has built up a tolerance for the drug through previous experience with it or with a related class of drug.

To what extent do the factors mentioned so far account for individual variability? Unfortunately, they only go a little way towards it, though they do give the psychopharmacologist some guide to the sort of variables that have to be controlled for in designing drug experiments. Even in the technically perfect or near-perfect experiment, however, there will still be a very wide range of response to the drug among the subjects taking part. These individual differences can be a nuisance, of course, if the investigator is trying to establish an average drug effect, though in recent years psychopharmacologists have become more interested in them for their own sake. It is becoming more and more obvious that most of the variation observed among people taking drugs is due to intrinsic differences in their psychological, or more strictly I should say their psychophysiological, make-up.

Although systematic investigation of this idea is only just beginning, the notion is really a very old one. Even in the late nineteenth century one French doctor wrote with confidence [23]:

It is a well-established notion that all subjects do not offer the same susceptibility to the action of medicaments and poisons. In respect of alcohol, Lasègue has specially insisted upon the differences of aptitude for intoxication: he remarked that if there are insusceptibles to alcohol there are also those, on the contrary, who are extremely susceptible to it, and suffer very rapidly its sad effects; they are alcoholizable.

Who, however, *are* the 'alcoholizables'? Most of the research on this problem has been founded on another everyday observation, namely that susceptibility to drug effects is in some way related to personality. Several people have put forward this view, including the famous psychologist William McDougall. In the nineteen-twenties he voiced what has been the most popular hypothesis, namely that, in the case of alcohol at least, it is the introvert who is most resistant, extraverts being the ones who 'suffer very rapidly its sad effects'. In more recent years a similar theory has been proposed by Professor Eysenck who has suggested that introverts have a greater tolerance of all depressant drugs but are more affected by stimulants than extraverted people. Eysenck has based his views partly on those of the Russian physiologist Pavlov who, like most scientists working with drugs, noticed considerable variability in the response of dogs during conditioning experiments. Pavlov was particularly interested in the effects of caffeine and, to account for the individual variation in response to this drug, he proposed that there were different 'types' of nervous system which corresponded to differences in temperament. Eysenck has applied a modern version of this nervous-type theory to man in order to explain why introverts and extraverts differ in their reactions to drugs.

There are several ways in which the psychopharmacologist can study the relationship between personality and drug response. One way is to administer a standard dose of some psychotropic drug, assess its effects by means of a number of psychological and physiological tests, and then see whether individual differences on these measures are related to scores on personality rating scales or questionnaires. In a series of studies of this kind an American psychologist, DiMascio, and his colleagues have isolated two broad personality types who differ in their response to a variety of psychotropic drugs. These have been named Type A and Type B personalities, respectively. People of Type A are described as practical, sociable and assertive extraverts with low anxiety and athletic body build. Type B people, on the other hand, are of slender body build, are more introverted and obsessional, have high anxiety and tend to inhibit rather than express their feelings.

In one of his early experiments DiMascio studied the response of these personality types to two different kinds of tranquillizer, phenyltoloxamine and reserpine [38]. All of the subjects were given a battery of psychomotor tasks, including serial addition, tapping, and a test of visuomotor coordination. Physiological reactions to the drugs were measured by recording changes in heart rate, respiration, skin temperature, and muscle tension. Overall the two drugs had somewhat different effects. Phenyltoloxamine had a sedative/hypnotic action, both on psychomotor performance and on subjective mental state. Reserpine had mainly physiological effects without altering task performance too much. The response to both drugs was different in the two personality types. In the case of phenyltoloxamine, Type A people showed greater hostility and more frequent negative attitudes to the drug situation, possibly because they found the sedating effects of this drug more unpleasant than Type B personalities, who described the drug effect as pleasantly relaxing. Task performance was also different in the two groups, Type A people improving and Type B people getting worse under phenyltoloxamine. The reaction to reserpine also differed in the two personality types. This time it was Type B individuals who expressed greater hostility, presumably because they found the physiological effects of the drug more unpleasant than Type A individuals. The differences in subjective feeling under reserpine were also reflected in the measures of autonomic activity, the physiological changes occurring in the two groups being in opposite directions. Thus the anxious introverted Type B personalities showed an increase in sympathetic predominance of the autonomic nervous system; whereas the more relaxed Type A personalities showed a decrease.

DiMascio and his colleagues have also demonstrated comparable differences in the response of their two personality types to other drugs, such as chlorpromazine and secobarbital. As in the experiment just described, the variations in subjective feeling produced by a drug are often revealed in the kind of physiological change that occurs. Since, as we have seen, this change may be in opposite directions in different people, it becomes important for the psychopharmacologist to identify different reaction-types if he is to avoid oversimplified generalizations about the physiological effects of psychotropic drugs. Some investigators, therefore, have approached the problem of individual differences from the other end, as it were, by selecting a number of 'physiological' types and seeing whether there is a variation in their drug response. In a study of this kind two Continental workers, Servais and Hubin, divided up groups of subjects on the basis of their autonomic nervous systems [55]. Following a traditional classification, they separated their subjects into three types. First, there were those who showed a relative predominance of the sympathetic division of the autonomic nervous system, whom they called sympathicotonics. A second group, named vagotonics, were characterized by relative predominance of the parasympathetic division. A third intermediate group showing stable autonomic balance without predominance of either division were called amphotonics. A comparison was then made of the response of these three types to amphetamine and to the tranquillizer, meprobamate. It was found that the two major types, sympathicotonics and vagotonics, differed considerably in their physiological reaction to both drugs. Whereas sympathicotonics showed a marked rise in pulse rate following the administration of amphetamine or meprobamate, the opposite was true of vagotonics, who reacted with a fall in pulse rate. The result for amphetamine is particularly interesting because it demonstrates that the rise in heart rate which is often said to occur with this drug is only true of certain people.

An important implication of this kind of experiment is that the *average* drug effect observed in a group of people will clearly be as much a function of the individual characteristics of the subjects making up the group as of the pharmacological action of the drug itself. Thus, if a particular personality or physiological type happens to predominate then the overall drug effect may be quite opposite from that observed in a sample made up of people of a quite different type. Sample variations of this sort probably account for the apparently contradictory results sometimes obtained with the same drug in otherwise identical experiments. These individual differences also emphasize how the psychopharmacologist has to look, not just at the overall effect of a drug, but at how particular individuals within his sample react to it. Occasionally, for example, he may find that a drug has apparently had no significant effect on the group as a whole and may be misled into thinking the drug is inactive. However, his measure of average change could well mask a genuine drug effect if different subjects within the group have responded in opposite directions. This is illustrated in another of DiMascio's experiments on personality and drugs [46]. There he studied the effects of three drugs on nonsense syllable learning. The drugs concerned were a sedative, secobarbital, and two tranquillizers, chlorpromazine and trifluoperazine. Compared with a placebo none of these drugs produced very much overall change in the learning scores of the group as a whole. However, when the subjects were divided up into Type A and Type B personalities, some marked drug effects appeared. As shown in Figure 6.3 the two personality types were affected in opposite ways. On all three drugs Type B people (anxious introverts) improved their learning scores, while Type A

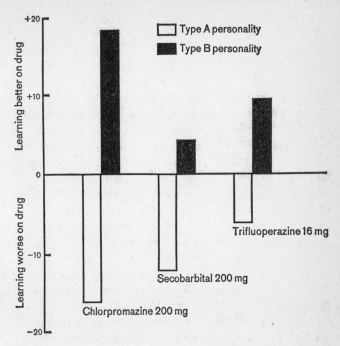

Fig. 6.3. Effects of three drugs on nonsense syllable learning in Type A (extravert) and Type B (introvert) personalities. Scores represent differences between drug conditions and an equivalent placebo condition. See text for further description of the two personality types.

(From an article by J. D. McPeake and A. DiMascio.)

people (relaxed extraverts) became consistently worse. Clearly these drug effects would not have been isolated if only the average changes in performance had been examined.

All of the experiments just described have been concerned with individual differences in the response to small single doses of drugs and the evidence suggests that the *way* a person reacts is related to his personality. What, however, about the *amount* of a given drug he can tolerate? To answer this question requires a rather different experimental strategy. Here, instead of giving the same dose of drug to everybody, what we need to do is to administer the drug in a progressive fashion and see whether some people are more rapidly affected by it than others. Put in this way the answer will, of course, almost certainly be 'yes'. What we really want to know is whether variations in susceptibility are a function of personality. The evidence suggests that they are, as is illustrated by the results of an experiment carried out some years ago at the Maudsley Hospital by Rodnight and Gooch [53].

Rodnight and Gooch were interested in the relationship in normal subjects between personality factors and susceptibility to the effects of nitrous oxide. The procedure adopted was to administer progressively increasing concentrations of nitrous oxide in oxygen to each subject while he performed alternately on two psychological tasks. The gas concentration was raised in a step-wise manner every five minutes. At each stage the subject carried out a simple pegboard test of finger dexterity followed by an arithmetical task in which he was required to double a short list of digits. As expected there were wide individual differences in the rate at which performance of both tasks became impaired. By calculating the slope of performance change on each test it was possible to derive two indices of each subject's susceptibility to nitrous oxide. These indices were then related to scores obtained from the Maudsley Personality Inventory which had previously been administered to the subjects and which gave measures of extraversion and neuroticism. These personality characteristics were chosen because, as discussed briefly already, there were some reasons for believing that extraverts, at least, would be more susceptible than introverts to the depressant effects of nitrous oxide. In fact, the results obtained were rather more complicated than that, though significant relationships with personality did emerge. Overall there was little correlation between drug tolerance and extraversion score, whichever index of gas susceptibility was used. Susceptibility was found, in fact, to depend on the degree of both extraversion *and* neuroticism.

Again this was true for both indices of susceptibility. Rodnight and Gooch demonstrated the interaction between extraversion and neuroticism in the following way. First they divided their whole sample of subjects into two halves: those with high and those with low scores on the neuroticism scale. They then separately correlated the indices of gas susceptibility with extraversion in the two halves. Next, correlations with neuroticism were calculated separately for two subgroups divided this time into high and low scorers on the extraversion scale. This analysis uncovered two highly significant relationships between personality and drug tolerance. One was that among subjects having a low neuroticism score it was the introverts who tended to be more susceptible to nitrous oxide. The second was that among the extraverts in the sample it was the more neurotic who were most susceptible. The greatest gas susceptibility was found in subjects who were both highly neurotic and highly extraverted. People of this type tend to be predisposed to hysterical and psychopathic disorders and it is interesting to note that neurotic patients actually diagnosed in that way also show very poor tolerance of depressant drugs, as I shall discuss in more detail later.

The technique used by Rodnight and her colleague has the advantages associated with nitrous oxide that were discussed in an earlier chapter. On the other hand, it has the disadvantage that the index of susceptibility it provides is rather cumbersome to compute. Other simpler methods of measuring an individual's drug tolerance have, therefore, been more popular among psychopharmacologists. All of these techniques have been developed and used mainly in a psychiatric setting. Since they will be discussed in detail in the next chapter, here I will only describe the principles behind them and the general use to which they have been put in studying variability of drug response among normal subjects. The procedures referred to all involve giving the subject a slow, continuous injection of a drug, usually a depressant, until some predetermined change in his behaviour occurs. The amount of drug injected up to that point, normally corrected for his body weight, then provides an index of his tolerance for the drug. Almost any easily recognizable and measurable alteration in the subject's response can be used as a criterion for assessing when he has reached his drug-tolerance threshold, as it is called. The most commonly used criteria are some change in the subject's brain-waves or autonomic nervous system, or a sudden change in his ability to perform a simple psychological task. An even simpler criterion, if a general depressant drug is being studied, is the point at which the person goes to sleep.

The use of these drug-threshold procedures in normal subjects has generally tended to confirm the findings obtained by Rodnight and Gooch with nitrous oxide. That is to say, the tolerance of other depressant drugs, such as the barbiturates, is related both to how extraverted the person is and to how much anxiety or neuroticism he displays. Thus, the anxious, introverted, obsessional individual will require much more barbiturate to reach a threshold of sedation than the extraverted and rather hysterical personality. The combination of extraversion and neuroticism is seen most clearly in neurotic patients themselves, who simply represent extreme forms of these two personality characteristics. It is not surprising therefore, to anticipate the next chapter a little, that clear differences have been found in the sedative drug tolerance of chronically anxious or obsessional neurotics and those with hysterical or psychopathic disorders. As we shall see there, the variability in tolerance of sedative drugs parallels a broad personality 'dimension' the opposite ends of which are occupied by these two neurotic types. Teasing out the relationships between personality and drug tolerance in normal subjects is rather more difficult because their behaviour is less extreme in all respects. Even so, work that has been carried out so far in this area of psychopharmacology indicates that a substantial part of the individual variability in response to drugs is due to personality factors, particularly those associated with introversion and anxiety. The relative importance of psychological, as distinct from purely physical, variables in determining drug susceptibility is well illustrated in a study recently carried out by a colleague, Dr Herrington, and myself. Over a number of years we have measured sedative drug thresholds in several hundred normal and psychiatric subjects. In calculating our index of drug tolerance we have always applied a correction for body weight to the amount of drug injected up to our chosen criterion of sedation. In this respect we have followed normal pharmacological practice, expressing the drug threshold, in this case for amobarbital, as an index of milligrammes of the drug injected per kilogramme of body weight, mg/kg for short. Quite recently, however, we examined the relationship between weight itself and the absolute, uncorrected amount of drug required to sedate different subjects. Rather surprisingly we found that, although heavier people did tend to take more of the drug, the correlation between weight and absolute amount was actually very small indeed. In fact, in some subgroups of our total sample the relationship was zero or even negative, more drug being required to sedate people who were lighter in weight. On the other hand, drug amount *was* correlated with personality measures and with various physiological measures which are themselves related to personality. Under the particular conditions of our experiments, therefore, a person's tolerance of drugs was much more a function of temperament than of tonnage! Of course, this may not be true in all situations in which drugs are administered. It may not be so, for example, where drugs are given by mouth in small doses or where some other feature of a drug's effect is measured, such as the rate at which an oral dose is absorbed or metabolized. Here, weight or some other physical factor related to it is probably as important. Nevertheless, the result provides a striking example of the major contribution of 'nervous type' to drug susceptibility.

If personality plays such an important role in drug response, how does this arise? To what extent, for example, does heredity determine individual differences in drug tolerance? Like the questions just posed, the answer to them is double-edged.

Knowledge of the genetic factors involved in the response to drugs would tell us something about the underlying mechanisms of drug action. At the same time it would also tell us something about the physiological and genetic basis of the personality characteristics that help to determine drug effects. Unfortunately, research on this aspect of human pharmacogenetics – as it is called – has scarcely begun. Most of the work has been concerned with pathological reactions to drugs: for example the abnormal sensitivity to barbiturates found in people suffering from the porphyrias, a group of rare metabolic diseases recently brought to fame as the probable cause of George III's madness.

The few studies of normal human subjects that have been carried out suggest that the individual's reaction to drugs may indeed be determined, to an important degree, by heredity. As in other genetic studies of human characteristics, the evidence is based on the investigation of twin pairs. One such study of a single pair of monozygotic or 'identical' twins, named Albert and Andrew, was described some years ago by Dr Glass in the United States [28].

Glass was interested to see how similar the twins were in their response to caffeine, which he administered in the form of five cups of strong coffee. The drug effect was measured by getting the twins to carry out a target-aiming task, in which they had to throw a 'dart' – actually a dissecting needle – at a number of small rings drawn on a sheet of paper. Each twin was given a series of trials on the test both with and without the drug. On the first occasion Albert performed under caffeine, while Andrew acted as his no-drug control. On the second occasion their roles were reversed. Figure 6.4 illustrates the twins' performance under each condition. It can be seen that they both responded to caffeine in a remarkably similar fashion, each showing exactly the same kind of performance curve when working under the drug. Dr Glass later confirmed this result in a more controlled experiment in which he used a lactose placebo and administered the drug to the twins, not as coffee, but as capsules of caffeine

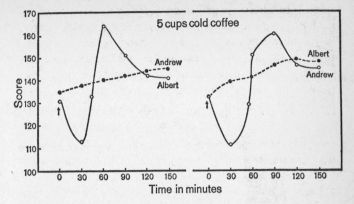

Fig. 6.4. Effect of caffeine on the performance of a target-aiming task in a pair of identical twins. Note the very close similarity in the performance curves (solid line) of the two twins after they had drunk five cups of coffee. Dotted lines represent performance on the same task under no-drug conditions.

(Reproduced by permission of B. Glass and Association for Research in Nervous and Mental Disease.)

citrate. The striking similarity in the drug response of the twins contrasts markedly with the great variability found by Glass in a randomly selected group of people whom he also tested under the same conditions. There the performance curves of different subjects varied so widely that he could observe no systematic effect of caffeine. Each person appeared to react to the drug in a manner peculiar to himself.

Convincing as they are, results from a single pair of twins are hardly conclusive. However, a more complete twin study carried out in our own laboratory by Dr Esther Ross and myself also supports the idea that the way a person reacts to drugs is determined very much by heredity. We have measured the tolerance of amobarbital in sets of twins, using one of the sedative drug-threshold procedures referred to earlier. Following the normal practice in this kind of work we compared a group of monozygotic, or one-egg, twins with a group of dizygotic, or two-egg, twins. If heredity plays an important part in drug response then monozygotic twins, being genetically identical, should require very similar amounts of drug to become sedated. Dizygotic twins, on the other hand, because they are no more alike than ordinary brothers and sisters, should differ very much more from each other. Figure 6.5 illustrates the results we obtained on eleven monozygotic twin pairs and ten dizygotic pairs. The diagram

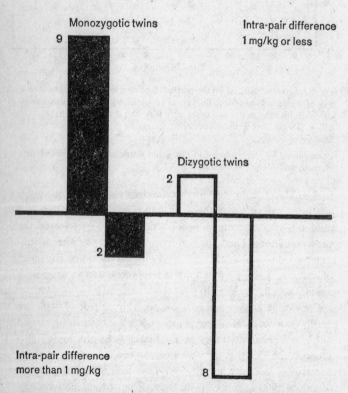

Fig. 6.5. Comparison of monozygotic and dizygotic twins on sedative drug tolerance test. Diagram shows the number of pairs in each group who differed by more than or less than 1 mg/kg in the amount of amobarbital required to sedate them.

shows the number of pairs in each group who differed from each other by more than or less than 1 mg/kg, a difference, incidentally, which represents a very small amount of drug indeed. It can be seen that most of the monozygotic twins showed differences of less than 1 mg/kg, some pairs actually having almost exactly the same tolerance thresholds. In contrast, the variation among dizygotic twins was much greater. All but two pairs differed by more than 1 mg/kg, while the average difference was nearly three times that figure.

As a general rule, then, the tolerance of sedative drugs seems to depend very much upon genetic factors. Of course, the results of the experiment just described were not perfect, some monozygotic twins being quite dissimilar in drug tolerance. How did this difference come about if they were genetically identical? It is impossible to say, though it is known that throughout development many influences operate to make monozygotic twins less rather than more alike, so that in research of this kind we are always underestimating the contribution of heredity to a particular characteristic. The fact that some apparently otherwise identical twins can differ does serve to emphasize, however, that all behaviour is the end-product of both heredity and environment, the latter including everything that happens to the individual from conception onwards. All that we can hope to do in twin research is to make a statistical estimate of the *relative* contribution of genetic factors. In the case of drug response heredity does appear to be especially important, despite occasional exceptions due to, as yet, unknown environmental influences.

The variations in drug response described in this chapter obviously make life rather difficult for the psychopharmacologist trying to reach some general conclusion about the effects of different psychotropic drugs. All that he can hope to do about such variation is to try and understand how it arises and then control for it in designing his experiments or hope that most of it will be cancelled out when different groups of subjects are being compared. If he is actually interested in variation for its own sake then life is still difficult, though never dull. The dependence of drug response on personality, for example, is an exciting fact, because it opens up an important way of examining the physiological basis of personality, one of the most difficult areas of behaviour to study scientifically. Here we have looked only at normal personality. However, some of the most valuable evidence in this particular branch of psychopharmacology has come from studying how the psychiatric patient reacts to drugs, a part of the story of individual variation that will be taken up in the next chapter.

Measuring Mental Illness with Drugs   7

To some readers the title of this chapter may seem a contradiction in terms. In one sense it is. The individual fears and anxieties of the mentally ill patient are so personal and grounded in his life-history as to defy precise measurement. Here, however, we shall be looking at mental illness in a slightly different way, viewing it as a biological disturbance and concerning ourselves, not with the content of the patient's illness, but with the processes underlying it. Such a view leads us to ask questions like 'What are the physiological correlates of the patient's anxiety or depression?' rather than 'What is he anxious or depressed about?' Neither approach to the problem is superior to the other, though, in principle at least, the processes of mental disorder are easier to quantify. This has certain advantages. If we could accurately measure the physiological disturbances that occur in different mental illnesses then we might be able to provide the psychiatrist with some objective procedures for classifying psychiatric patients and assessing the effects of treatment. There are few, if any, such procedures in everyday use in psychiatry at the present time. The psychiatrist is not in the happy position of his medical colleague who, in arriving at the diagnosis of a physical complaint, often makes use of various laboratory tests. Psychiatric diagnosis has to be made on the basis of the patient's superficial symptoms – except, that is, where the mental disturbance is secondary to some physical disease or where it results from gross damage to the brain. An intensive search is going on at the moment for objective physiological indicators both of neurosis and of the more severe mental disorders of depression and schizophrenia. Some of this experimental work involves the use of drugs and serves to illustrate how, at one level of behaviour, important features of mental illness can be measured.

In the case of mild mental disorder, such as neurosis, measurement with drugs is really a logical extension of the work discussed in the previous chapter. There we saw that the response to drugs depends to some extent on personality. It is not too surprising, therefore, to find that neurotic patients also differ among themselves in their reactions to drugs. The differences are clearly seen on the sedative drug tolerance tests already referred to. The principle behind these tests, it will be recalled, is that an estimate is made of the amount of drug required to produce a predetermined change in the individual's behaviour or physiological state. The first procedure of this type was described by Dr Shagass, a Canadian psychiatrist now working in the United States, who called his technique the 'sedation threshold test' [56]. As illustrated in Figure 7.1 Shagass used a twofold criterion to decide a person's sedation threshold. The main one was based on the effect of barbiturates on the electroencephalogram (EEG). If a drug such as amobarbital is injected intravenously and the brainwaves recorded from the frontal areas of the brain, it is found that certain fast waves – those between 15 and 30 cps – increase progressively in amplitude. The effect is shown in the left half of

Figure 7.1. The increase in amplitude can then be plotted as a function of the amount of drug injected. When this is done it is found that the amplitude curve rises gradually and then flattens out, as shown in the right half of the figure. This inflexion point, as it is called, occurs at different drug dosages for different people, and the amount of drug required to produce the effect in a given individual is regarded as his sedation threshold. Shagass also found that the sudden change in brain-wave amplitude coincided with the point where the person's speech became slurred and he used this sign as an additional behavioural criterion of the sedation threshold. As noted in the previous chapter, the sedation threshold itself is conventionally recorded as the amount of drug injected per unit of body weight, usually in mg/kg.

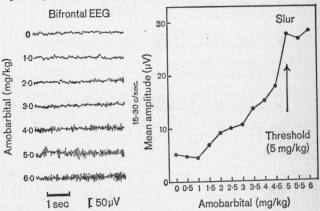

Fig. 7.1. Method of determining the sedation threshold from the electroencephalogram. On the left are shown successive samples from an actual EEG tracing recorded from the frontal areas of the head while a subject is receiving an injection of amobarbital. Reading downwards, it can be seen that, with increasing amounts of drug, there is a gradual rise in the amplitude of the faster brain rhythms. On the right, amplitude is plotted against drug dosage. Note the sudden change in amplitude at – for this subject – about 5 mg/kg, the point taken as his sedation threshold.

(Reproduced by permission of C. Shagass and the publishers, *Psychosomatic Medicine*.)

Using this technique Shagass determined the sedation threshold in several hundred neurotic patients [57]. His results are shown in Figure 7.2, which illustrates, for different types of neurosis, the relative proportion of patients with sedation thresholds falling below 3.5 mg/kg and above 4.0 mg/kg. It can be seen that the

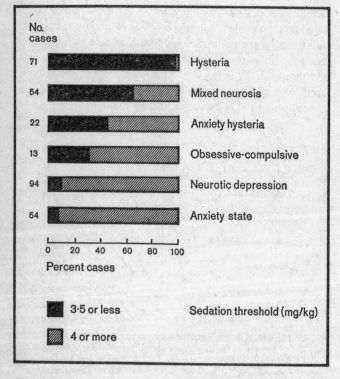

Fig. 7.2. Diagram showing the relative frequency with which patients with different types of neurotic disorder have either low or high sedation thresholds. Compare particularly the preponderance of high sedation thresholds in patients with anxiety states and the low thresholds found in almost all of the hysterics.

(Reproduced by permission of C. Shagass and the publishers, *American Journal of Psychiatry*.)

sedation threshold was low, that is the tolerance of barbiturates was poor, in almost all patients diagnosed as hysterical neurotics. This group included people of histrionic personality as well as those with dramatic physical symptoms, like paralysis or blindness, that were entirely due to psychological causes. At the other extreme were patients suffering either from chronic anxiety or from a neurotic form of depression that could be traced to some environmental stress.

Soon after Shagass introduced his EEG technique, several other methods for determining the sedation threshold were developed. One simple procedure, based on behavioural rather than brain-wave changes, was devised some years ago by Dr Herrington and myself [13]. We hit on the idea of getting the subject to do a simple arithmetical task while he was having the injection of amobarbital. What we did was to play a tape-recording of random digits occurring at the rate of one every two seconds. The subject simply had to multiply each number by two, a procedure which allowed us to monitor the drug effect continuously. The injection proceeded at a constant rate until the subject failed to double ten consecutive digits. His performance on the task could then be plotted in the form shown in Figure 7.3 and from this we could work out the sedation threshold. As seen in the diagram, the absolute values of sedation threshold determined by this method were somewhat greater than those obtained by Shagass using his EEG technique. This is because in all cases more drug is required to bring about a change in observable behaviour than to produce a detectable alteration in brain-waves. However, the important point is that the *relative* differences in sedation threshold among various neurotic groups are the same whichever method is used. Figure 7.3 shows the sedation threshold curves for just three individuals, but when Dr Herrington and I compared groups of subjects we found, like Shagass, that hysterics as a whole tended to show the poorest drug tolerance. The highest sedation thresholds were again found in dysthymics, a general term used to cover all introverted

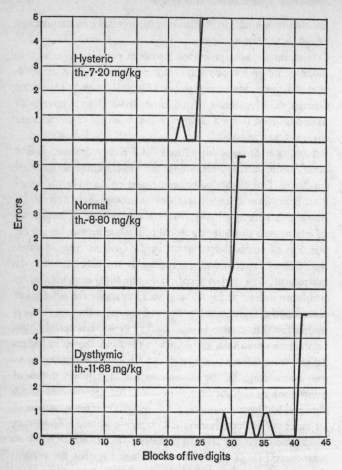

Fig. 7.3. Performance curves for three individuals, illustrating the digit-doubling method of determining the sedation threshold. The curves represent the number of errors made in each block of five digits, the injection of drug being stopped when five errors have been committed in two consecutive blocks. The amount of drug required to produce this effect is then calculated in the form of a sedation threshold, as shown on the right of each curve.

(Reproduced by permission of the publishers, *Journal of Mental Science*.)

neurotics who suffer from chronic anxiety, obsessional symptoms, or neurotic depression.

Of course, the arbitrary division of neurosis into two or more discrete sub-types is only a matter of convenience. In practice the different forms merge into one another, as shown in Figure 7.4. There it can be seen that, despite the fact that there is a significant difference in the *average* sedation thresholds of dysthymics and hysterics, the distribution of scores within the two groups overlaps considerably. In other words, there is a continuous variation of sedation threshold, forming a symmetrical distribution similar to that found for other behavioural characteristics like intelligence. This continuum of drug tolerance seems to be a sort of physiological counterpart of a personality dimension, the extreme ends of which are defined by dysthymic neurotics, on the one hand, and hysterical neurotics on the other. In general, normal people tend to fall in the middle of the continuum, though as it happens this was not true in the particular sample of normal subjects shown in Figure 7.4. In their case, although the average sedation threshold was slightly higher than the mean for hysterics, a large proportion of the subjects in the group tended to have generally low thresholds. There was a good reason for the bias towards low, rather than high, sedation thresholds in this particular normal sample. As part of our research we had given personality questionnaires to all our subjects and when we looked at the scores in the normal sample we found that the group was made up largely of neurotic extraverts. In other words, they were mainly people predisposed to hysterical reactions and therefore of a type who would be expected to have low sedation thresholds. Perhaps people like that are more likely to volunteer – or more easily persuaded – to have an injection. In any event if we had taken a more representative group of normal individuals their sedation thresholds would probably have overlapped about equally with those for the two extreme neurotic groups.

The personality continuum that coincides with variations in drug tolerance has, for obvious reasons, been named dysthymia-

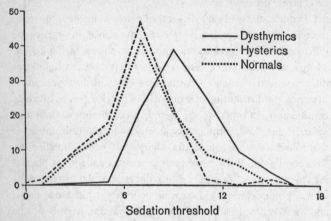

Fig. 7.4. Frequency distribution of sedation threshold in three groups of normal and neurotic subjects. Note the overlap between the groups and the continuous variation from high to low sedation threshold.

(Reproduced by permission of Pergamon Press Ltd.)

hysteria or obsessionality-hysteria. So far we have looked at the continuum mainly from the point of view of differences that are found between groups of patients diagnosed according to the kind of neurotic symptoms they show. A more direct way of examining it, however, is to see whether there is any relationship between drug tolerance and the particular characteristics associated with obsessionality and hysteria. In another of his experiments Dr Shagass did just that [58]. Using his EEG method Shagass determined sedation thresholds in over 200 neurotic patients. Two psychiatrists rated the patients for the presence or absence of obsessional and hysterical traits. A single score of obsessionality-hysteria was then calculated for each patient. The relationship between this score and sedation threshold over the whole group is shown in Figure 7.5. It can be seen that with increasing sedation threshold there is a progressive increase in obsessionality-hysteria rating; the greater the tendency towards

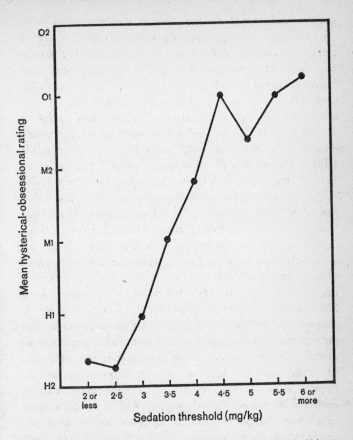

Fig. 7.5. Diagram illustrating how the variation in sedation threshold is related to hysterical (H) and obsessional (O) traits of personality.

(Reproduced by permission of C. Shagass and the publishers, *Journal of Nervous and Mental Disease.*)

obsessionality, rather than hysteria, the higher the sedation threshold tends to be.

Terms like 'dysthymia', 'hysteria', and 'obsessionality' refer very much to the kinds of symptoms found in neurosis and the question that arises is how these findings in neurotic patients link up with those on drug tolerance and personality in normal people. For example, how far does the sedation threshold measure basic personality traits and how far does it reflect some temporary feature of neurotic illness? The answer is that it probably does both. As far as basic personality characteristics are concerned there is evidence that the dysthymic-hysteric continuum just described is a composite one made up of the two personality dimensions of introversion and neuroticism. As we saw in the previous chapter these two dimensions interact in a complex way to determine drug tolerance in normal individuals. The different neurotic types really represent extreme examples of this interaction and allow us to recognize the broad continuum of dysthymia-hysteria that parallels the full range of drug tolerance. On the other hand, the hospitalized or outpatient neurotic is not *just* someone a bit further along the continuum than most of us, a kind of less than normal 'normal'. He is marked off from the rest of the population by virtue of the fact that he, or someone close to him, is sufficiently worried to seek psychiatric help. He is, if only temporarily, suffering from some degree of psychological imbalance, such as an exacerbation of an unwanted neurotic habit or an increase in his anxiety above its usual level. It would not be too surprising if this temporary change in behaviour were reflected in an alteration in his psychophysiological state as measured by tests like the sedation threshold. In one of his many experiments Shagass showed, in fact, that improvement and deterioration in the neurotic patient's condition were both accompanied by changes in the sedation threshold [59]. Figure 7.6 illustrates the kind of result he obtained in one of his patients, a woman suffering from chronic anxiety. Shagass tested the patient's sedation threshold repeatedly during periods of worsening and remission of her symptoms. It can be seen that on occasions when her anxiety appeared to have been alleviated the sedation threshold went down, only to rise again when her anxiety symptoms increased.

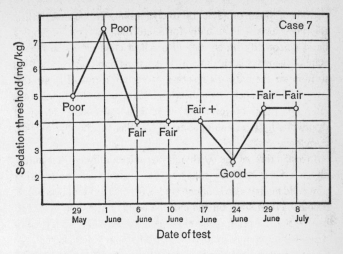

Fig. 7.6. Fluctuations in the sedation threshold of a chronically anxious patient, showing how the threshold rose markedly when her emotional state was rated as 'poor' and fell again as her anxiety symptoms diminished.

(Reproduced by permission of C. Shagass and the publishers, *Journal of Psychosomatic Research*.)

These shifts in sedation threshold contrast markedly with results obtained in normal people where the measure has been found to remain remarkably constant over relatively long periods of time. Do they not contradict the impression given so far that drug tolerance is a fairly permanent correlate of personality, possibly having a strong genetic basis? Not really, because no human characteristic is entirely immutable in that sense. A good non-psychological example is that of body build. Whether one is long and thin or short and round depends very much on heredity and, once established, the basic proportions do not alter much. However, certain measures of body type such as weight or amount of fat deposited will fluctuate from time to time. Usually the change is fairly slight but may be significantly greater during periods of illness or addiction to cream buns. In the case of drug tolerance tests it is actually fortunate that, as well as tapping basic personality traits, they also reflect changes in the mental state of the psychiatric patient. This means that they can be used to monitor the patient's response to certain forms of treatment. An example of such an application of drug tests will be described later on. First, however, let us look a little more closely at dysthymia-hysteria and at some of its other psychophysiological correlates.

Investigation of the dysthymia-hysteria continuum has naturally not been confined solely to the measurement of sedation threshold but has also included studies of other kinds of behaviour, such as performance on some of the tasks of attention described in Chapter Three. For example, it has been shown that, compared with hysterics, dysthymic neurotics maintain their vigilance better on tasks requiring sustained attention. They also take fewer rest pauses, work more rapidly on simple motor tasks, and condition more quickly. This all adds up to the picture of the dysthymic individual as someone in a chronically high state of alertness or arousal – hence, of course, the greater amount of barbiturate required to sedate him. By comparison even with normal individuals the hysterical neurotic is poorly aroused. This difference between the two personality types is reflected in their respective levels of anxiety. The dysthymic's characteristically high anxiety level contrasts markedly with the hysteric's abnormal lack of anxiety, an unconcern about his condition which some of the early French psychiatrists labelled *belle indifférence*. These differences in anxiety-proneness are themselves reflected in variations in the activity of the autonomic nervous system. Thus, the dysthymic is autonomically very responsive and reacts strongly to stimulation with sweating, raised heart rate and other signs of increased activity in the sympathetic nervous system. In the same situation the hysteric tends to show a rather sluggish sympathetic reaction. How do these differences in autonomic responsiveness tie in with the variation in drug tolerance found among dysthymics and hysterics? We might expect, for example, that people with high sedation thresholds would also be those who have very reactive sympathetic nervous systems. One way of finding out would be to correlate the sedation threshold with a measure of how different people react to mild psychological stress. Some years ago we did this in our own laboratory by recording the heart rates of dysthymic and hysterical neurotics while they were performing on a vigilance task. As predicted, we found that patients with high sedation thresholds had higher heart rates during performance than those with low sedation thresholds.

An alternative and rather more direct way of tackling the same problem is to use another type of drug test. Over the years a number of drug techniques have been specially devised to measure the reactivity of the autonomic nervous system. The principle behind these techniques is fairly simple. A drug is injected which has its main action on the autonomic system. The response to the drug is measured by recording the physiological change that occurs, usually in blood pressure. Since the autonomic system is dedicated to maintaining equilibrium in the body, the blood-pressure change will quickly be counteracted by homeostatic mechanisms and the blood pressure eventually restored to normal. The immediate response to the drug and the speed with which equilibrium is regained will vary widely from one person to the next and the 'profiles' of blood-pressure change found have been used to try and distinguish different autonomic reaction types. Equilibrium is maintained in the autonomic system by virtue of the opposing action of its sympathetic and parasympathetic divisions, the former predominating during emotional arousal and the latter during relaxation and sleep. In theory, therefore, four kinds of drug can be used, corresponding to their actions of either stimulating or inhibiting one or other half of the autonomic system. Thus, epinephrine produces the familiar racing pulse by stimulating the sympathetic system, which in turn triggers off restraining influences from the parasympathetic division. Other drugs, however – like atropine – block the para-sympathetic system, but some of its effects, such as widening of the pupil, are similar to those caused by direct sympathetic stimulation. If we wish to study sympathetic reactivity as such then the best choice of drug is from the other two types, that is either parasympathetic stimulators or sympathetic blockers. Both kinds of drug induce a physiological state – e.g. a fall in blood pressure – which stimulates the sympathetic nervous system to restore equilibrium. The speed at which this happens or some measure correlated with it can then be used as an index of sympathetic reactivity.

In the particular example to be mentioned a sympathetic blocking drug, called phentolamine, was used in order to see whether people with high sedation thresholds show a brisker or greater subsequent rise in blood pressure than those with low sedation thresholds [17]. The drug was injected intravenously and the patient's blood pressure measured repeatedly throughout the test. As expected, the average pattern of response was an initial fall in blood pressure, then a rise. However there was tremendous variation among different individuals, as shown in Figure 7.7, which illustrates some typical blood-pressure profiles. Four subjects – two neurotics and two normals – are included in the diagram, together with the values for their sedation thresholds. The first point to notice is that the two neurotics, on the right and left, showed by far the most extreme reactions to the drug; but they did so in quite different ways. The patient on the right showed a big fall in blood pressure which returned to normal very slowly, suggesting a sluggish sympathetic reaction to the drug. It will be seen that his sedation threshold was rather low. By contrast, the other patient who had a high sedation threshold reacted with a very strong sympathetic response. His blood pressure fell very little and on recovery actually rebounded well beyond what it was before the drug was injected. These two extreme reaction profiles are replicated in a diminished form in the two normal subjects shown in the middle of the diagram.

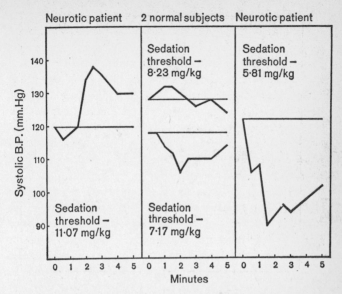

Fig. 7.7. Typical blood-pressure curves in four subjects given phentolamine. Note the more extreme, though opposite, reactions of the two neurotic patients and the tendency for the patient with a high sedation threshold to show a predominant rise and the patient with a low threshold to show a predominant fall in blood pressure. Similar, but smaller, responses are shown by the two normal subjects.

(Reproduced by permission of the publishers, *British Journal of Psychiatry*.)

Again, however, it was the subject with the lower sedation threshold whose blood pressure recovered more slowly. The other subject, in fact, showed no fall that could be measured; only a small rise.

How does the apparent relationship between these two quite different drug tests hold up over a group of subjects? Figure 7.8 shows the result of plotting the sedation threshold against the changes in blood pressure, measured as the relative amount of rise or fall. It can be seen that with increasing sedation threshold there is a progressive tendency for rises, rather than falls, in blood

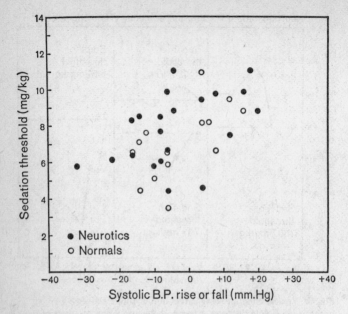

Fig. 7.8. Relationship between sedation threshold and change in blood pressure after phentolamine in a mixed group of normal and neurotic subjects. Note the orderly tendency for subjects with high sedation thresholds to show rises, and those with low thresholds to show falls, in blood pressure on the phentolamine test.

(Reproduced by permission of the publishers, *British Journal of Psychiatry*.)

pressure to occur. In other words, the higher a person's sedation threshold the more reactive is his sympathetic nervous system; or, in everyday terms, the more likely is he to show strong physiological signs of anxiety under stress. This was true in normal subjects as well as in neurotic patients, suggesting that the difference between them is quantitative, rather than qualitative. Here again, then, we find that personality variations in dysthymia-hysteria have a physiological counterpart in drug response.

So far we have been concerned with the way the immediate

response to an acute dose of drug given by injection is used to determine the physiological state of the neurotic patient. A logical extension of this, but a slightly different problem, concerns the assessment of the effect of a drug given to a patient as part of his or her treatment. Here, of course, the drug will be administered orally in a small dose over an extended period of weeks or months; though the drug itself may be the same or one similar to that used in the estimation of the sedation threshold. Alternatively, it may be a non-barbiturate tranquillizer. In either case we would expect some change to occur in the patient's physiological reactions, especially if he reported feeling subjectively better. We could actually use the sedation threshold – or some similar drug test – to assess the improvement, as Shagass did with his neurotic patient described earlier. However, in this situation other methods are equally applicable, as Lader and his colleague Lorna Wing demonstrated in a recent study at the Maudsley Hospital [41]. In an earlier experiment, by measuring heart rate, galvanic skin response and other autonomic functions, Lader and Wing had confirmed that anxiety neurotics are physiologically more reactive than normal people. The next step in their research was to see whether the same patients would become autonomically less reactive – and subjectively less anxious – after a short course of treatment with a sedative. All of the patients spent a week on a placebo and a week on the active drug, amobarbital, the sequence in which the two treatments were given of course being varied in different individuals, so as to allow for an order effect. Measurements of autonomic function and ratings of subjective state were made at the beginning and end of each treatment. Figure 7.9 illustrates the results for one of the physiological measures used, the number of spontaneous fluctuations in galvanic skin response, an index of anxiety or arousal we came across earlier, in Chapter Three. It can be seen that, compared with the placebo condition, the active drug caused a marked reduction in the patients' physiological arousal. What about their subjective feelings? The most obvious changes concerned physical

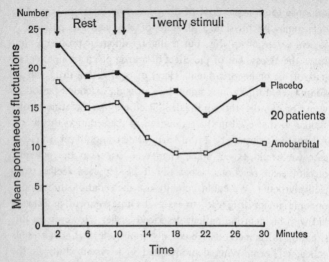

Fig. 7.9. Measuring the effects of treatment with a sedative drug in twenty anxious neurotic patients. A comparison is made of the mean number of spontaneous GSR fluctuations found after a period on placebo and a period on the active drug. In each case measurements were made over a thirty-minute session, first with the patient at rest and then under conditions where auditory stimuli were played at random intervals.

(Reproduced by permission of M. H. Lader and the Institute of Psychiatry, London.)

symptoms of anxiety, such as shakiness and palpitations, which were significantly reduced. Rather less change occurred in 'psychological' anxiety, such as feelings of wanting to avoid fear-provoking situations. This last finding illustrates, incidentally, that drugs are valuable for treating neurosis only if they are combined with some attempt to treat the patient's specific symptoms, either by psychotherapy or by conditioning methods. The experiment as a whole, however, illustrates how it is possible to quantify the effect of drugs on the physiological processes underlying neurotic symptoms.

Let us turn now to a rather different problem of measurement in psychiatry, namely that of depression. Of all the symptoms complained of by the mentally ill patient depression is certainly the most common. A melancholic mood can, of course, accompany any mental (or physical) illness. As a psychiatric diagnosis, however, depression refers to the condition in which the change in mood forms the major part of the patient's psychological state. In reality the term covers a rag-bag of conditions and, in order to classify them, psychiatrists have sometimes found it useful to distinguish two types of depression. The first type, called neurotic or reactive, describes the kind of depression which can be accounted for in terms of some stress in the patient's environment. The second type, called psychotic or endogenous, comes out of the blue and appears to occur independently of the patient's life experience. As with other disorders of the personality the boundary between these two types of depression is blurred and it is not always easy for the psychiatrist to put patients into one or other category on the basis of their symptoms alone. Yet it may be important to try and do so since it is usually agreed that one of the most widely adopted treatments for depression, electroconvulsive therapy or ECT, is more effective in the psychotic than in the neurotic form of the illness. The psychiatrist would be greatly helped therefore if he had available objective measuring instruments that would enable him to diagnose the different types of depression and consequently to select the appropriate kind of treatment suited to each patient. Although we are still a long way from this happy state, at an experimental level some progress at least has been made as a result of research using techniques like the sedation threshold.

Most of the experimental evidence about neurotic, reactive depression shows that patients suffering from this condition are basically of dysthymic personality. Studies of the sedation threshold have tended to confirm this. A glance back at Figure 7.2 (page 150) illustrates that in Shagass's original study of different types of neurosis, his neurotic depressives generally had high sedation thresholds, being very similar in this respect to patients suffering from anxiety states. In a special study of depression as such, Shagass then went on to show that psychotic depressives, on the other hand, tended to have low sedation thresholds [57]. His results, gathered on over 200 depressive patients, are illustrated in Figure 7.10. There it can be seen that,

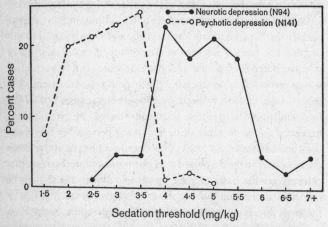

Fig. 7.10. Frequency distributions of sedation threshold in two types of depression, showing how neurotic depressives tend to have high and psychotic depressives low sedation thresholds.

(Reproduced by permission of C. Shagass and the publishers, *American Journal of Psychiatry*.)

although there is some overlap, the two kinds of depression are well separated on the sedation threshold.

Shagass and his colleagues next asked themselves whether the sedation threshold could pick out those patients who would respond best to electroconvulsive treatment. On the basis of what is known about the better response of psychotic depressives to ECT they predicted that patients with low sedation thresholds would improve more after this form of treatment than those with high sedation thresholds. At the end of their courses of treatment all depressed patients receiving ECT were rated for degree of improvement. They were divided into three groups, those showing marked, those showing moderate, and those showing little or no improvement in their depression. These categories of improvement were then related to the sedation thresholds obtained before treatment had begun. The result of the experiment is shown in Figure 7.11, where it can be seen that Shagass's prediction was confirmed. As expected, the sedation threshold was closely correlated with the amount of improvement expected after ECT. The higher the sedation threshold the less chance there was that the depressed patient would respond favourably to this treatment.

If the sedation threshold can help to select depressed patients for suitable forms of treatment, it is reasonable to ask whether the test can also be used to assess changes in mental state on recovery from depression. Earlier in the chapter we saw that the sedation threshold can alter as a patient gets more or less anxious. Does this also apply to depression and, if so, what sort of changes occur in depressed patients after treatment? A recent study by Dr Perez-Reyes and his colleagues at the University of North Carolina goes some way towards answering these questions [50]. Their work is also of special interest because they used a new method of measuring sedative drug tolerance, a procedure they called the 'GSR-inhibition threshold'. This technique makes use of the effect of barbiturates on the galvanic skin response. The reader will recall from Chapter Three that one of the effects of intravenous barbiturates is to abolish spontaneous fluctuations in skin resistance as the subject becomes more and more drowsy. Another, parallel, change that occurs is a reduction in the size of GSRs given to specific stimuli applied at intervals during the injection. Since individuals differ in the amount of drug required to abolish the GSR altogether, it is possible to exploit the effect as a way of measuring drug tolerance. What Perez-Reyes did was to inject thiopental sodium while the subject listened to sets of three digits read out at twenty-second intervals. The GSR-inhibition threshold was then taken as the point at which the digits failed to elicit a galvanic skin response.

In his study of depression using this technique Perez-Reyes

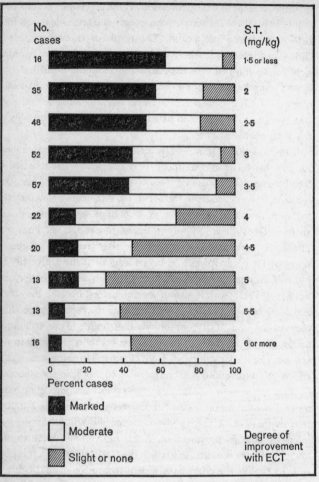

Fig. 7.11. Relationship between sedation threshold and the degree of improvement found in depressed patients after electroconvulsive treatment. As the sedation threshold increases so the likelihood of a good response to ECT diminishes.

(Reproduced by permission of C. Shagass and the publishers, *American Journal of Psychiatry*.)

measured the GSR-inhibition threshold in three groups of people, neurotic depressives, psychotic depressives, and normal subjects. All subjects were tested twice, with an interval of about a month between the two tests. During this interval all of the patients received appropriate treatment for their depression. Figure 7.12 shows the results of the experiment. It can be seen

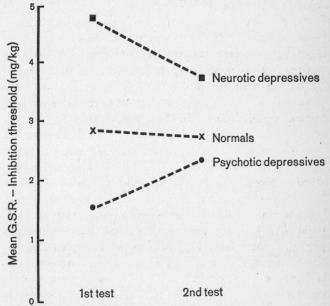

Fig. 7.12. Diagram illustrating the 'normalizing' effect of treatment on the GSR-inhibition threshold of depressed patients. After treatment (second test) the mean threshold of psychotic depressives rose; that of neurotic depressives fell.

(From an article by M. Perez-Reyes. Reported here by permission of the author.)

that on the first testing, before any treatment had been given, the mean GSR-inhibition threshold in psychotic depressives was very much lower than it was in neurotic depressives, thus confirming Shagass's conclusion that drug tolerance is quite different in the two types of patient. More interesting, however, are the results obtained on retesting the subjects. Normal subjects, who of course received no treatment, showed little change, indicating that in the absence of any marked alteration in psychological state the measure is very stable. Both depressed groups, on the other hand, showed a considerable change in threshold, though in opposite directions. Thus, the thresholds of psychotic depressives went up; those of neurotic depressives went down.

The picture that emerges, then, from the studies just described is of two forms of depression which are physiologically distinct and which respond in different ways to treatment. Neurotic or reactive depression seems to be another form of dysthymic neurosis in which the tolerance of sedative drugs is very high. Like other dysthymics, these patients seem to be in a state of high central nervous arousal, the effect of treatment being to make them less aroused. The psychotic or endogenous depressive, on the other hand, is someone who is extremely sensitive to barbiturate effects, but who becomes less sensitive when he recovers. How do the results obtained in psychotic depressives accord with the observation that patients of this type respond better to electroconvulsive therapy? In order to answer that we really need to know more about how ECT works. One hypothesis to explain its effects is that ECT has a central stimulating action on the brain, causing an increase in sympathetic reactivity. This explanation is an attractive one for two reasons. First of all, as we shall see in the next chapter, it fits in quite well with what is known about the neurophysiological basis of the sedation threshold; namely, that it appears to measure the activity of those parts of the brain which help to maintain arousal and sympathetic reactivity. Secondly, it is known that, as well as having low sedation thresholds, depressives who respond to ECT also show sluggish sympathetic reactions to autonomic drugs of the kind described earlier. So it might be expected that a stimulating effect of ECT would produce most improvement in those patients who are initially rather poorly reactive.

Of course, none of this tells us much about the exact nature of psychotic depression or why ECT is such a successful treatment for the condition. As we have seen, poor sympathetic reactivity – and low sedation thresholds – are also found in other psychiatric patients who are not depressed: hysterics, for example. The main value of the drug techniques described is that they perhaps help to provide a more objective way of classifying different types of depression. That, at least, takes us one step nearer the understanding and rational treatment of these disorders.

Let us turn finally to the most bewildering jigsaw in psychiatry, namely schizophrenia, or to put it more correctly, the schizophrenias; for this is not a single disorder but a conglomeration of different reaction types, almost as varied as the personalities in which they occur. Frequent failure to appreciate this fact, even by expert research workers in the field, is probably one reason why we have made so little progress in understanding the nature of the schizophrenias. Thus, a good deal of research effort – and money – has been expended in looking at the chemistry of the brain for some single underlying 'cause' of schizophrenic illness. The search is likely to be about as fruitful – or fruitless – as the quest for the philosophers' stone. For it is now clear that the schizophrenias are a group of very complex personality disorders the causes of which are unlikely to be revealed until we know very much more about the intricate biological and social influences that mould normal behaviour. This is not to belittle the value of biochemical and neurophysiological research in this area, but only to emphasize that its contribution to our understanding of the schizophrenias will only be as great, or as small, as its contribution to our understanding of normal psychology. Research into the schizophrenias is, of course, proceeding on a broad front, ranging from the biochemical to the social, and work on behavioural drug response represents only a tiny fraction of the total research output. It will, nevertheless, help to illustrate one of the ways in which the research scientist is trying to make some sense out of these puzzling disorders. First, however, let us take a closer look at the nature of the problem itself.

Three difficulties are common to all research into schizophrenia. The first arises from the fact that there is no real agreement about what group of symptoms constitutes a schizophrenic disorder. Many experienced psychiatrists claim that they know by intuition and may (successfully) diagnose it, though usually more by 'smell' than by logic. Most would agree that it involves an extensive disintegration of the personality in all its spheres, social, emotional, and intellectual. However, total agreement on more precise criteria than this is lacking and use of the term 'schizophrenic' may vary widely from one country or one clinic to the next. A patient diagnosed as schizophrenic by one psychiatrist may be regarded by another as hypomanic, psychotically depressed, or neurotic. This difficulty alone makes the comparison of different experiments in the area rather hazardous.

The second difficulty is that the personality changes associated with schizophrenia do not follow an easily predictable course. They may occur insidiously over many years and without any clear beginning or in a series of acute breakdowns which push the individual a little further each time towards social and emotional deterioration. In either case the drift into a chronic state will be accompanied by widespread physiological and psychological changes which will, in turn, be reflected in any experimental measure the research worker cares to take. The early and late phases of the schizophrenic reaction probably represent different conditions, and conclusions drawn about one may not be applicable to the other. The picture may be further complicated by any physical treatments, such as drugs, the patient has received in the past. As we shall see later, these may drastically alter the very measures we are using to try and describe the underlying disorder.

The third difficulty has already been touched upon, namely the variety of ways in which the schizophrenias present themselves. Traditionally they have been divided into four broad types: paranoid, hebephrenic, catatonic, and simple. In the paranoid form the patient's thinking is dominated by delusional ideas, mainly of being persecuted; though in other respects his personality may be remarkably well preserved. The hebephrenic, on the other hand, shows gross disorganization of personality, bizarre language and thinking, and fatuous or incongruous emotional response. In catatonia the patient withdraws from human contact into a state of physical immobility and posturing sometimes punctuated by outbursts of aggressive excitement. The fourth, simple, type is characterized by slow deterioration of social and personal habits, frequently reflected in a drift into vagrancy. As pure forms these different types are rarely seen and in practice they usually merge one into the other. Their range serves, however, to underline the fact that we are not dealing with a single illness, but with a number of quite different reactions.

Faced with such a complex problem how can the research worker reduce it to manageable proportions? Part of the answer is by carefully selecting the patients he chooses to study, making sure that he controls for such factors as the length of time they have been ill and the kind of treatment they have received. Having done this he can then proceed in one of two ways. One way is to narrow down on some single well-defined feature of schizophrenic behaviour and try to understand it by manipulating it experimentally. Let us look at an example of this particular approach.

As we saw a moment ago, in the catatonic form of schizophrenia the patient actually withdraws physically from reality and enters a state of stupor in which he appears to be completely unresponsive to those around him. To the casual observer it seems as though his whole nervous system is in a state of very low arousal akin to sleep. However, physiological recordings taken from patients in catatonic stupor have quite clearly demonstrated that, on the contrary, they are very *highly* aroused; one might almost say they are hyper-alert. In keeping with this dissociation between overt behaviour and internal physiological state it has been found that catatonic patients respond in a paradoxical way to sedative drugs. In one such experiment catatonics were given injections of amobarbital and at the same time recordings were made of EEG activity, muscle tension, and heart rate [66]. The results of the experiment, which are illustrated in Figure 7.13,

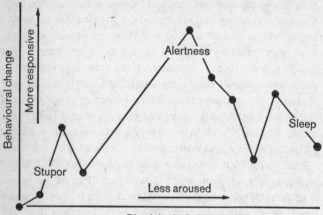

Fig. 7.13. Diagram illustrating the paradoxical alerting effect of a sedative drug in patients with catatonic stupor. As the drug made them physiologically less aroused, so they became behaviourally more responsive. This effect was followed, at higher doses, by a normal drift into sleep.

(From a diagram by J. M. Stevens. Reproduced by permission of the publishers, *Psychosomatic Medicine*.)

showed that physiologically the drug caused the usual shift down the sleep-wake continuum. Behaviourally, however, it caused the patients to become much more active to begin with, many of them emerging completely from their catatonic stupor. When the injection was continued beyond this point the stupor did not return. Instead the patient simply went to sleep.

This experiment is one of a number which have shown that often the behaviourally least responsive or withdrawn schizophrenics may actually be physiologically the most highly aroused. One explanation suggested for this curious reversal of the normal state is that in the schizophrenias there is a defect in the regulating mechanisms which control sensory input into the nervous system. As we saw in Chapter Five this may be experienced subjectively by the patient as a feeling of stimuli 'rushing in' on him from all directions. It has been argued that, in order to cut down sensory input to a minimum, the catatonic patient withdraws into immobility even though he remains – as some recovered catatonics have indeed reported in retrospect – highly alert to changes in the environment. What actually happens in the brain itself is, of course, not known, though one possibility is that a state of what Russian physiologists have called 'protective inhibition' is induced, whereby the nervous system responds to the increased sensory input with massive inhibition, thus protecting itself from overstimulation.

In experiments of the kind just described the investigator tries to bring under control a limited aspect of schizophrenic behaviour, selecting patients who show the characteristic in question and studying how it changes under different conditions. The second kind of research strategy to be mentioned has the slightly different aim of trying to establish differences between different kinds of schizophrenia, usually by relating some experimental measure or combination of measures to important clinical features of the illness. The purpose here is to try and give some account of the variability of the schizophrenias. To illustrate this method let us look at some recent work on the sedation threshold.

Earlier we saw that an important factor determining the schizophrenic patient's behaviour is the length of time he has been ill. It is now fairly certain that whatever physiological changes occur when the schizophrenic first breaks down, these do not persist unaltered if he proceeds to become more chronically ill. Instead the nervous system seems eventually to readjust in the same way that the patient's overt behaviour readjusts, leaving him with only the residual, or what have been called the 'burnt out', signs of the original acute breakdown. These changes from the acute to the chronic phases are reflected in the sedation threshold [57]. Thus, although by no means true of all patients, the sedation threshold in acutely ill schizophrenics is generally rather low. In chronic patients, on the other hand, it tends to be much higher. Furthermore, as shown in Figure 7.14, there is an

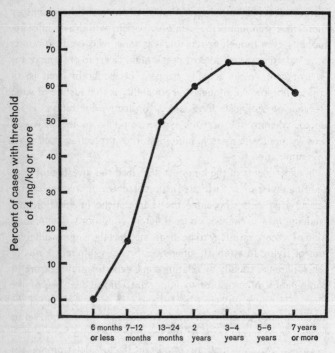

Fig. 7.14. Relationship between sedation threshold and duration of psychotic symptoms, plotted as the percentage of schizophrenic patients at different stages of their illnesses with thresholds of 4 mg/kg or above. Note the sharp rise during the first two years of schizophrenia.

(From a diagram by C. Shagass. Reproduced by permission of the publishers, *American Journal of Psychiatry*.)

orderly relationship between the sedation threshold and the length of time the patient has had his schizophrenic symptoms. As the interval since the first breakdown increases so the sedation threshold rises progressively up to a peak of between one and two years, after which it levels off. This result confirms the idea that the early and late phases of the schizophrenic reaction are physiologically quite distinct conditions; or, to put it more precisely, as one phase merges into the other, so the physiological state alters.

From the point of view of prevention, diagnosis, and treatment the more important problem to be solved is what happens in the early stages of the schizophrenias, when the initial change in personality occurs. Unhappily, by itself the sedation threshold can tell us very little since, as we have already seen, at least two other psychiatric disorders – hysteria and psychotic depression – are also characterized by low sedation thresholds. And in any case, although on average the sedation thresholds of acute schizophrenics are low, there is still considerable variation from one patient to the next. This variation does not show any simple relationship with the type of schizophrenic reaction. Does this mean that the sedation threshold simply measures some rather non-specific feature of psychiatric illness? Or does it mean that, as in psychotic depression, the changes associated with it *are* significant but that they only represent one part of a more complex disturbance of the central nervous system in the schizophrenias? Recent research on the test has suggested that the latter may be more true, and that when used in combination with other experimental measures the sedation threshold may tell us more about the nature of the schizophrenias than was at first thought.

Some years ago, in the early 1960s, Dr Shagass and his colleague Dr Krishnamoorti, then working together in Iowa, and Dr Herrington and myself, working here in Britain, independently discovered a rather curious fact about the sedation threshold in schizophrenic patients [30; 40]. Unbeknown to each other, we were both doing research on the relationship between the sedation threshold and other experimental tests in different kinds of psychiatric illness. We had both focussed attention on one particular measure, the rather odd visual illusion called the Archimedes spiral after-effect which I described in Chapter Five. It will be recalled that this test involves measuring the strength of the visual illusion of after-movement which follows previous fixation of a rotating black spiral. We were interested in the test as another measure of central nervous arousal in different personality types. As predicted, we found that dysthymic neurotics had much stronger and more persistent after-effects than hysterical neurotics. This, of course, fits in quite nicely with the differences found between these patients on the sedation threshold, and indeed over the whole group of neurotics there was a significant positive relationship between the sedation threshold and the Archimedes spiral after-effect. In general the higher the sedation threshold the longer the after-effect tended to be. However, when we looked at the same two tests in schizophrenic patients, both Shagass and Krishnamoorti and Dr Herrington and myself found that this relationship no longer held. Instead, the opposite was true! As shown in Figure 7.15, schizophrenics with high sedation thresholds unpredictably had very short spiral after-effects, whereas those with low thresholds had long after-effects. Consequently the correlation between these two measures was the other way round from that in neurotic patients. Thus it was not the absolute difference on either test that distinguished between neurotics and schizophrenics, but the relationship between the two measures.

Subsequently we ourselves examined this peculiar finding in more detail, looking to see if performance on the sedation threshold and spiral after-effect was related in any way to such factors as the type of schizophrenic breakdown, the presence of certain kinds of symptom and so on. We did this by dividing the schizophrenic group into two halves; those with high sedation thresholds and short spiral after-effects, and those with low thresholds and long spiral after-effects. When these two subgroups were compared on a number of characteristics they were found to correspond roughly with two broad clusters of schizophrenic

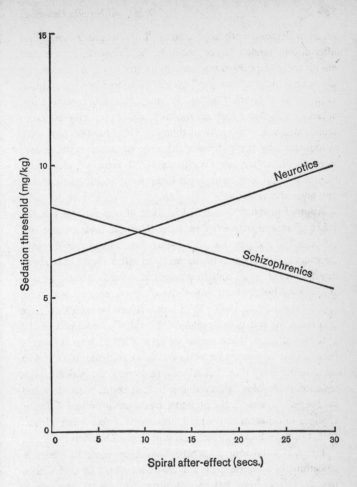

Fig. 7.15. Comparison of neurotic and schizophrenic patients on the sedation threshold and the Archimedes spiral after-effect. Results are shown as average trend lines representing the way the measures relate together in each group. The performance of neurotics is exactly as predicted, long visual after-effects being reported by patients with high sedation thresholds, and vice versa. Reversal of this relationship in schizophrenia is paradoxical, but may represent a 'dissociation' of arousal mechanisms in the nervous systems of schizophrenic patients (see text).

reaction. Patients with high sedation thresholds and short spiral after-effects tended to be sociable, behaviourally active and emotionally responsive but were more frequently paranoid and disordered in their thinking. Those in the low sedation threshold, high spiral after-effect group, on the other hand, were slow, socially withdrawn and emotionally 'flat', and suffered more from emptiness or poverty of thought. These relationships were complicated by the additional influence of factors such as age, intelligence, and basic personality – all three of which undoubtedly help to determine the form the schizophrenia takes in any given individual.

Another problem we studied in some of our patients was the effect of treatment on the sedation threshold and spiral after-effect. All of our patients were in their first schizophrenic breakdown and so it was possible to test them before they had received any treatment at all and then again afterwards. Retesting was confined to those patients who showed a good recovery from their illness. Figure 7.16 shows the results. It can be seen that after treatment the sedation thresholds and spiral after-effects of the patients shifted so that over the group as a whole the relationship between the two measures was once more reversed. Now it was no different from that normally found in neurotic patients, high sedation thresholds again going with long spiral after-effect and vice versa. As seen in the diagram, treatment produced different changes in different individuals, the overall effect being a complex, but nevertheless orderly, shift in the two measures.

The odd behaviour of schizophrenics on these two tests is something of a puzzle, especially as we have little idea what tests like the spiral after-effect are measuring. In general, however, it is beginning to look as though the altered relationship between the sedation threshold and spiral after-effect may reflect a peculiar kind of disturbance of the attention and arousal mechanisms discussed in the earlier chapters of the book. There we saw that attention to the environment involves both a general alerting response and a more specific scanning or filtering of stimuli

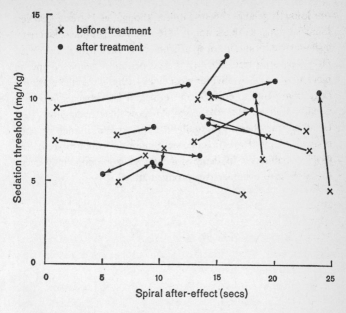

Fig. 7.16. Diagram showing the shifts in score on sedation threshold and spiral after-effect in individual schizophrenic patients after treatment. Note that after treatment the relationship between the two tests is restored to that found in neurotic patients (cf. Figure 7.15).

(Reproduced by permission of Pergamon Press Ltd)

entering the nervous system, the two processes normally being nicely in tune. It seems as though in the schizophrenias – and perhaps under LSD – the same two mechanisms may get out of step or their functions in some way become naturally dissociated from each other. If such a change did occur then the effects on the personality would be catastrophic and mental life a chaos – as indeed it is in these conditions. Interestingly enough, whatever the disturbance is it appears to take a different form in different individuals, a fact which confirms the considerable variability observed in the behaviour of schizophrenic patients.

The results I have just described take us almost to the edges of our knowledge about mental illness, though, as I stressed earlier, there is a considerable amount of research being undertaken from a similar viewpoint, if not specifically concerned with drug effects. However, drug research in this field perhaps occupies a special place because of its obvious close links with the parallel quest for drug treatments to control severe mental disturbance. We have already seen how, in the case of neurosis, both diagnosis and treatment may benefit mutually from research in human psychopharmacology. Though immensely more difficult problems, the psychotic illnesses of depression and schizophrenia may eventually yield to a similar two-pronged attack.

Drugs, Behaviour and The Brain   8

So far we have seen how psychotropic drugs can be used experimentally to analyse various aspects of human behaviour. What do these experiments tell us about the brain mechanisms involved? Or, put another way, how far is it possible to link up the behavioural effects of drugs with what is known about their action on the central nervous system? The ideal way to answer these questions would be to observe an individual's behaviour while under the influence of a drug and at the same time record the changes that are occurring in different parts of his brain. However, that would mean putting electrodes inside the brain itself, a procedure to which most volunteers for human drug experiments would object! So the psychopharmacologist has to go about the task in a more devious way. He naturally relies to a considerable extent on animal experiments where a drug's effect on the brain can be studied more directly. This method clearly has certain limitations, an obvious one being the difficulty of generalizing from animals to humans. Another arises from our present ignorance about the exact mechanisms of drug action, even in the animal brain. Thus, interpreting the results of an experiment on the neurophysiological effects of a drug may often be just as much a matter of inspired guesswork as the interpretation of its effects on behaviour. In practice relating these different kinds of evidence together advances, as in most scientific research, by a series of approximations to the truth. This involves looking, first of all, for superficial similarities in the behavioural drug response of animals and humans. Inferences drawn about brain activity from human drug studies can then be checked against facts obtained from actual experiments on the brain in animals. By a constant exchange of information among different branches of psychopharmacology it gradually becomes possible to piece together some of the events linking a drug's action on the brain with its effects on behaviour.

Although the human psychopharmacologist cannot actually record from inside his subjects' skulls, he can go some way towards bridging the gap between the brain and behaviour. As we have seen elsewhere, he has at his disposal a number of physiological techniques, such as the galvanic skin response and the electroencephalogram, which enable him to take, admittedly rather crude, soundings of what is going on in the nervous system. He can, for example, fairly accurately monitor some of the simpler changes produced by psychotropic drugs, such as alterations in a person's level of alertness. From his observations using these techniques he may deduce that the drugs concerned affect certain brain mechanisms which, as we shall see later, may be pinpointed more exactly by parallel experiments on animals. The most direct indicator of brain activity available to the human psychopharmacologist is the electroencephalogram or EEG and in the previous chapter we saw how brain-wave changes can be used to monitor the effects of large doses of barbiturates administered during the determination of drug tolerance thresholds.

Even so, as used there the EEG is a rather limited procedure – in fact not much better than the galvanic skin response – and, unless the changes in psychological state are very gross, simple inspection of the EEG tracing can tell us little about the subtler aspects of brain activity. However, progress in the field of electronics is now making it possible to extract more precise information from the EEG. This is beginning to provide the psychopharmacologist and other behavioural scientists with more sophisticated tools with which to explore the human brain.

One important advance is the development of a method of EEG analysis called 'averaging'. Prior to the introduction of this technique it was difficult, if not impossible, to detect in the EEG anything other than a gross change in the brain's response to stimulation. Suppose, for example, we want to measure the brain's reaction to a very brief light stimulus flashed in a subject's eyes. It would not be feasible to do so by just looking at the ordinary EEG tracing. This is because the change in brain rhythm following the stimulus will be of very small amplitude and have a rather complex wave-form. As shown in Figure 8.1, it would be 'lost' against the high amplitude background activity that makes up the normal EEG. However, suppose we keep delivering light flashes to the subject's eyes – say, a hundred of them, one at a time every few seconds. As we have seen, the responses to individual flashes will be undetectable. But imagine superimposing upon one another the EEG tracings following each flash of light. The random background activity will begin to cancel out, leaving behind only the wave-form common to the light stimuli themselves. The more tracings we add to the pile the clearer the wave-form will become, or, more technically, the higher will be the signal-to-noise ratio. The characteristic brain wave that emerges is called the 'average cortical evoked response', also known simply as the evoked response or evoked potential. Extracting it from the EEG record by hand, according to the method described, would be very tedious, of course, and rather inaccurate. In practice, therefore, the whole procedure is carried out by computer which samples the EEG record for a set period of time, say 500 milliseconds, following each stimulus. By summating the amplitude of the EEG for successive milliseconds of all samples the wave-form of the evoked response is compiled electronically and then converted into a visual plot.

The shape of the evoked response varies from one sense modality to another, being different for auditory compared with visual stimuli. The general wave-form, however, is that shown in Figure 8.1, where it can be seen that the response is made up of several component waves. The first three of these are known as the primary complex and the second group – numbered 4 to 7 in

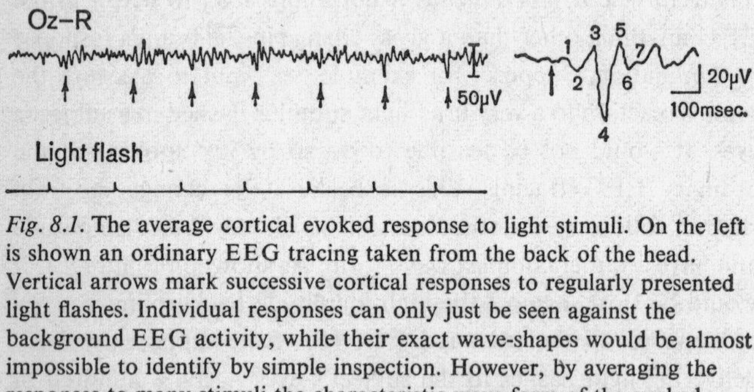

Fig. 8.1. The average cortical evoked response to light stimuli. On the left is shown an ordinary EEG tracing taken from the back of the head. Vertical arrows mark successive cortical responses to regularly presented light flashes. Individual responses can only just be seen against the background EEG activity, while their exact wave-shapes would be almost impossible to identify by simple inspection. However, by averaging the responses to many stimuli the characteristic wave-form of the evoked potential, shown on the right, can be reconstructed. See text for discussion of the numbered components of the evoked response.

(Reproduced by permission of G. Corssen and the publishers, *Anesthesiology*.)

the diagram – as the secondary complex. Following the secondary complex a further series of rhythms, called the afterdischarge, can also be recognized. The various components of the evoked response are known to alter according to the subject's mental state, the onset of sleep, for example, being associated with a reduction in the size of the primary complex and a corresponding increase in the secondary complex. Study of the evoked response by psychopharmacologists has demonstrated that different psychotropic drugs may also alter its wave-form [15].

Figure 8.2 shows the effect of giving a subject an intravenous injection of the barbiturate, secobarbital, compared with two placebo injections of dextrose and saline. Neither of the latter treatments had any effect on the evoked response. The active drug, however, produced changes somewhat similar to those of normal sleep. The primary complex was markedly reduced in size while the secondary complex – especially wave 4 – became progressively larger. Corssen and Domino, who carried out this experiment, also studied the effects of giving subjects injections of chlorpromazine. That drug produced rather different changes in

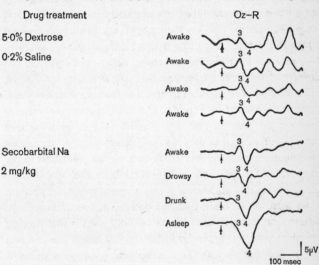

Fig. 8.2. Comparison of the effect of a barbiturate and two placebo injections on the visual evoked response. Vertical arrows mark the onset of the light stimuli. Note particularly the progressive increase in the size of component 4 under the active drug.

(Reproduced by permission of G. Corssen and the publishers, *Anesthesiology*.)

the evoked response. The secondary complex was still increased in size, though less so than with secobarbital. The most obvious difference, however, was in the primary complex, the amplitude of which remained quite unchanged even after the drug had sent the subjects to sleep.

These changes in brain activity fit in quite well with what is known about the behavioural effects of psychotropic drugs. The reader will recall from Chapter Three that one of the main differences between tranquillizers and sedative/hypnotic drugs is that the latter have a general depressant effect on psychological performance. By comparison, tranquillizers like chlorpromazine are rather more selective in their action. The changes in evoked response reflect this difference, chlorpromazine affecting only certain components and the barbiturate producing a more typical sleep-like pattern. Can we deduce anything more precise about where in the brain these two types of drug are acting and how they produce their different effects on behaviour? Probably not directly at the moment because neurophysiologists are not yet quite clear what significance to attach to the various components of the human evoked response. However, research on animals does suggest that the reason tranquillizers and sedatives have different effects is that they act on different parts of the brain's alerting mechanisms. I shall come back to this point later in the chapter, but first let us take a look at the brain itself, particularly at those areas that are known to play a crucial role in drug action.

An area of the brain that has become of special interest to behavioural scientists over the past twenty years is that running upwards from the lower brainstem to just below the cerebral cortex (see Figure 8.3). This is because it contains within it circuits that are essential to the brain's normal waking activities. The 'area' is actually a dense network of nerve fibres forming several interconnected functional systems. That part lying within the midbrain itself has been called the *ascending reticular activating system*, or ARAS for short. A continuous stream of impulses passes upwards from the ARAS to the cortex, toning it up and preparing it to respond to environmental stimuli. It is partly from here that variations along the behavioural sleep-wake continuum, described in Chapter Three, originate; the changes in GSR and

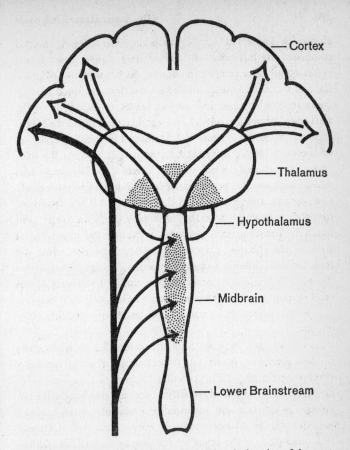

Fig. 8.3. Schematic diagram of the brain showing the location of the mesodiencephalic reticular system. The lower hatched area is the midbrain portion, the *ascending reticular activating system*; the upper hatched area is the *diffuse thalamic projection system*. The relative position of the hypothalamus is also shown. The bold black arrows illustrate the dual route by which sensory information travels through the brain, going both directly to the cortex and indirectly via the mesodiencephalic system.

other peripheral responses being external signs of what is happening in the brain. In animals the activating properties of the ARAS can be demonstrated by stimulating it directly through electrodes implanted in the midbrain. The sleeping animal stimulated in this way will immediately waken and become behaviourally more active. In addition, its brain waves will show signs of increased arousal, the large slow rhythms found in sleep being replaced by fast low voltage waves characteristic of the alert state. Above the ARAS is a second circuit called the *diffuse thalamic projection system*. This is situated in the diencephalon, or 'between-brain', so-called because it falls between the mid-brain, or mesencephalon, and the cerebral hemispheres. This thalamic system also activates the cortex but does so more selectively and for briefer periods of time than the ARAS. One of its functions is believed to be that of helping the brain to shift and focus its attention, thus probably providing the physiological basis of the attention-span changes discussed earlier. Both the thalamic and midbrain systems – sometimes known collectively as the mesodiencephalic system – come under the control of the cerebral cortex, which can either excite or suppress their activity. In addition, each has its own in-built excitatory and inhibitory circuits.

Extensive research in psychopharmacology has shown that the mesodiencephalic system is an important site of action for many psychotropic drugs which, according to chemical type, may damp down, excite, or selectively modify its activity, thus producing the changes in alertness and attention we notice subjectively and can measure with behavioural tests. Of course, this does not mean that other parts of the brain are immune to drug effects. On the contrary, many neural circuits will be affected, involving all areas of the brain, from the cortex downwards. One way of demonstrating the relative importance of different areas is to combine the administration of a drug with surgical procedures which, in animals, can isolate selected parts of the brain. A typical experiment will help to illustrated how this is done. The particular study to be described is also of interest because it provides a good example of how animal experimentation can complement parallel research in human psychopharmacology. The study was carried out by Dr Perez-Reyes, the originator of one of the drug threshold procedures discussed in the previous chapter. It will be recalled that his technique for measuring drug tolerance – the GSR-inhibition threshold – involved measuring the amount of thiopental sodium required to abolish an individual's galvanic skin response. Following his work with human subjects, Perez-Reyes took his research a stage further in order to try and specify the brain mechanisms responsible for the GSR-inhibition threshold. Before describing the experiment itself let us look briefly at the arguments behind it.

Animal research has demonstrated that the sweating of the skin which forms the basis of the GSR is controlled by several neural loops or circuits in the brain. Some of these send excitatory impulses and others inhibitory impulses to the skin, the GSR normally being the result of an interplay between activity in all of the circuits involved. Roughly speaking, the excitatory and inhibitory circuits can be identified with different anatomical levels of the brain. The main excitatory area is in the midbrain, in the region of the ARAS, and includes the hypothalamus, the central powerhouse of the autonomic nervous system. Below and above this area lie two inhibitory circuits, one in the lower brain-stem and the other in the cerebral cortex, which has a powerful restraining influence on the midbrain. The purpose of Perez-Reyes's experiment was to determine which of these circuits is most important in determining the GSR-inhibition threshold. The general argument was that thiopental has a progressively descending action on the brain, starting with the cerebral cortex. Thus the drug's first effect will be to remove the inhibitory influence of the cortical centres that damp down the GSR.* As

* Incidentally, if this is correct, an early sign of the drug's action should be an *increase* in GSR, a change actually noticed by Perez-Reyes while determining the GSR-inhibition threshold in human subjects. A more everyday example of the same phenomenon is the apparent tendency for small amounts of alcohol to have a stimulant effect. This, too, has long been ascribed, if rather more vividly, to the loosening of higher mental faculties and the release of more primitive centres in the brain.

more thiopental is injected, however, its effect will spread down-wards and the GSR-inhibition threshold will be reached, it was argued, just at the point where excitation from the midbrain centres is eliminated. At this point the inhibitory circuit in the lower brainstem, that is *below* the midbrain, should still be active, if indeed the middle excitatory areas are the main site of action of thiopental.

To demonstrate that this is so Perez-Reyes carried out an experiment on cats, who were of course fully anaesthetized throughout the whole procedure [50]. He recorded skin resistance from the animals' paws, using brief electrical pulses to elicit GSRs at regular intervals. An injection of thiopental sodium was continued until the GSR disappeared and the animal had reached its 'GSR-inhibition threshold'. Then the brain was transected at the top of the spinal column, an operation which removed the influence of the lower inhibitory centres. In all cases the GSR immediately reappeared, suggesting that before surgical transection these centres had still been active, and supporting the idea that the main effect of the drug was to damp down the midbrain excitatory centre. By inference, the GSR-inhibition threshold could be regarded as a measure of the strength of excitation in this area of the brain.

What are the implications of experiments of this kind for the studies of human drug tolerance described in the previous chapters? First of all they allow us to say something about the biological basis of personality and why it is that people respond differently to drugs. For example, we can infer that the mid-brain mechanisms controlling central excitation are probably especially active in introverted, anxious individuals compared with personality types who are more affected by sedative drugs. So the notion of 'nervous types', discussed in Chapter Six, starts to take on some physiological reality. In the case of psychiatric illness we can begin to specify which brain mechanisms may be disturbed in different types of patient, as well as throw light on how and why different treatments work. A good example is that already discussed in the previous chapter, namely the changes brought about by electroconvulsive therapy in psychotically depressed individuals.

Actually in a sequel to the experiment just described Perez-Reyes went back to test out on humans the conclusions that he had drawn about the brain mechanisms involved in the GSR-inhibition threshold [50]. He argued that if one temporarily raised the level of excitation in normal human subjects, then the tolerance of thiopental ought to be increased. What he did, therefore, was to assess the GSR-inhibition threshold in individuals who had previously been given an injection of methamphetamine, which he assumed would increase central excitation. The same subjects were also tested, for comparative purposes, after a saline placebo injection. The results were as predicted, the amount of thiopental required to abolish the GSR being significantly greater after methamphetamine than after saline.

A further extension to the experiment just described would, of course, be another animal study to see whether the amphetamines do increase excitation by acting on the midbrain. As a matter of fact there is already evidence that they do. In a series of investigations carried out at Birmingham University Professor Bradley and his colleagues have studied how a number of psychotropic drugs, including amphetamine, affect the excitability of the midbrain in cats. In the first group of experiments each drug's effect was measured by determining the amount of stimulation required to alert the animal at different dose levels [7]. Bradley used two methods of arousing the animals during the experimental sessions. One was by direct electrical stimulation of the midbrain reticular system in which an electrode had previously been implanted. The other was by means of an auditory stimulus played through a loudspeaker situated near the animal. In both cases the intensity of stimulation was gradually increased in small steps until an arousal response occurred. The criteria for deciding when the animal was aroused was based on changes both in brain-waves and in behaviour. It was considered that EEG arousal had occurred when fast low-voltage rhythms appeared in the electrocorticogram, a recording similar to the electroencephalogram except that it is taken, not from the scalp, but from the surface of the brain itself. Behavioural arousal was defined by the opening of the eyes, movement of the head, and contraction of the nictitating membrane, the third eye-lid vestigial in man but present in the cat. The intensity of stimulation required to produce these changes provided a measure of the animal's 'arousal threshold', which could then be plotted against increasing dose of each drug.

Figure 8.4 shows what happened with amphetamine. It can be seen that this drug caused an overall lowering of the arousal

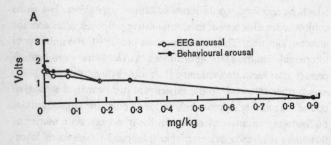

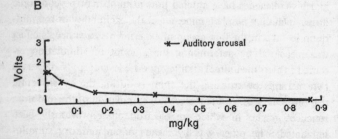

Fig. 8.4. Effect of amphetamine on the arousal response in cats. As the dose of drug increases so the strength of stimulation required to alert the animal diminishes. *A* represents changes in arousal threshold for direct stimulation of the brain and *B* the change in threshold for an auditory stimulus.

(Reproduced by permission of P. B. Bradley and Little, Brown and Co.)

thresholds, that is a reduction in the intensity of stimulation required to alert the animal. This excitant effect, which increased as a function of dose, was true both for EEG and behavioural arousal, whether induced by an auditory stimulus or by direct stimulation of the reticular system. The results therefore supported the idea that amphetamine increases the excitability of the midbrain areas, making them more sensitive to stimulation.

What about the effects of other drugs? As we might expect from Perez-Reyes's experiment, barbiturates have the opposite effect. Professor Bradley actually studied pentobarbital but found that, like thiopental, it had a marked dampening effect on the midbrain centres. Thus, in contrast to amphetamine, it caused a considerable rise in the arousal thresholds, both for auditory and direct electrical stimulation. However, the most interesting findings concerned two other drugs that were studied, namely LSD and chlorpromazine. In both cases the drug effect was confined to changes in the arousal response to the *auditory* stimuli. As can be seen in Figure 8.5, LSD greatly reduced the arousal thresholds for this kind of stimulation, but when the midbrain was stimulated directly the threshold for arousal remained unchanged. Effects of a similar kind, though of course in the opposite direction, were found with chlorpromazine. Even large doses of that drug produced relatively little change in the response to brain stimulation, though quite small amounts made the animal unreactive to sound stimuli. Here, then, we see how some of the behavioural effects of LSD and chlorpromazine are reflected in their action on the brain. Although the two drugs are, respectively, excitant and depressant, the *way* they produce their effects is quite different from that of ordinary stimulants and sedatives. Bradley concluded, in fact, that while amphetamines and barbiturates act directly on the midbrain reticular system, LSD and chlorpromazine alter the individual's arousal indirectly by making him more or less sensitive to information coming into the nervous system from outside.

In a further group of experiments Professor Bradley's research

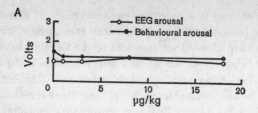

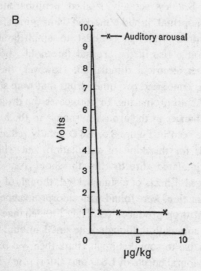

Fig. 8.5. Effect of LSD-25 on the arousal response in cats. Note how the amount of stimulation required to alert the animal is unchanged when the brain is stimulated directly (*A*) but falls sharply when an auditory stimulus is used (*B*).

(Reproduced by permission of P. B. Bradley and Little, Brown and Co.)

team has followed up this idea that chlorpromazine and LSD act specifically by altering the organism's sensitivity to its environment. In one study, carried out by Dr Key, recordings were made from the brain of a cat placed in different environmental surroundings [35]. The cat had an electrode permanently implanted in its dorsal cochlear nucleus, a relay station along the route from the ear to the auditory receiving area in the cortex. The electrical activity of the cochlear nucleus was monitored by measuring the amplitude of consecutive brain potentials evoked by high-frequency tones played at regular intervals. The animal was tested under two environmental conditions: while in a sound-proofed box and after being transferred to the noisier open laboratory. These conditions were alternated, an injection of LSD being given after the first three control sessions. The results of the experiment are illustrated in Figure 8.6. The most impor-

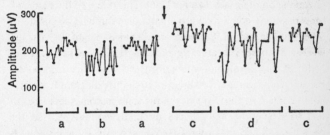

Fig. 8.6. Effect of LSD-25 on the fluctuation of the evoked response under different environmental conditions. The first three control periods were alternately under quiet (a) and noisy (b) conditions. Injection of the drug (arrowed) had little effect on the evoked response under quiet conditions (c), but produced marked fluctuations under noisy conditions (d).

(Reproduced by permission of B. J. Key and the *British Medical Bulletin.*)

tant effect to notice is how the amplitude of the evoked response became more variable when the animal was placed in the open laboratory. This was true even before the drug was administered (compare a and b in the diagram), but became much more marked under LSD (compare b and d). Now, it is known that the amplitude of the evoked response fluctuates much more if the stimuli around the animal have significance for it. So Dr Key was able to conclude that LSD had the effect of increasing the number of stimuli to which the animal was responding. The effect could only appear, of course, in varied surroundings where many stimuli were impinging on the brain; hence the smaller fluctuations found in the sound-proofed box.

Like the first experiment, this study was concerned with changes recorded in the brain. What evidence is there that the animal's *behaviour* reflects the increased sensitivity to stimulation apparently produced by LSD? In other experiments Bradley and his colleagues have taken the next logical step of studying cats in various learning situations arranged so as to test the hypotheses derived from their studies of the brain. In one such experiment Dr Key compared the effects of chlorpromazine and LSD, making use of a technique based on the well-known learning phenomenon of 'generalization' [36]. This refers to the tendency for a response, conditioned to a particular stimulus, to spread to other similar stimuli. Suppose an animal is taught, say, to lift its paw whenever it hears a tone of a particular frequency. It will be found that the animal will perform the same learned response, though less vigorously, when tones of slightly different frequency are presented. As the frequency of the tones becomes less like the one to which the animal was originally conditioned, so the response will become progressively weaker; or, if the response is an all-or-none affair, so the probability of it being evoked will diminish. Key argued that, if LSD were having the effect he supposed, then it should increase the amount of generalization that occurred during conditioning. Chlorpromazine, on the other hand, should *reduce* generalization, since its effect on the brain seems to be opposite to that of LSD. As shown in Figure 8.7, Dr Key's experiment confirmed these hypotheses. It can be seen that, although generalization occurred under all conditions its amount depended on the drug administered. While under LSD the animals made many more generalized responses even to tones very remote in frequency from the original conditioning stimulus. Chlorpromazine, on the other hand, had the effect of severely limiting the number of stimuli to which the animals responded. These results were interpreted in the following way. It was sug-

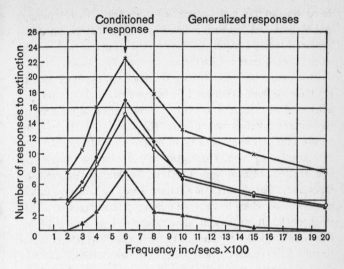

Fig. 8.7. Effect of LSD-25 and chlorpromazine on the amount of generalization occurring during conditioning. The top curve is for LSD, the bottom one for chlorpromazine, and the middle two for saline control testings. The vertical scale represents the strength of the animals' responses, both to the original conditioning tone (arrowed) and to tones of similar frequency. Note how, compared with placebo conditions, LSD increases and chlorpromazine decreases the strength of responses to tones distant in frequency from the original conditioning tone.

(Reproduced by permission of B. J. Key and the publishers, *Psychopharmacologia*.)

gested that conditioning and generalization can both be regarded as processes whereby the organism attaches meaning to stimuli that are previously neutral for it. It could be concluded, therefore, that under LSD stimuli take on greater significance than usual, while under chlorpromazine the opposite occurs.

Even this experiment is, of course, far removed from the psychiatric clinic or the psychedelic den. Nevertheless, we can see some similarities in the behaviour of Dr Key's cats and that of humans given the same drugs. Subjectively chlorpromazine makes the psychotic patient more indifferent to his surroundings.

In contrast to this, a characteristic feature both of schizophrenia and of the model psychosis induced by LSD is that the individual becomes unduly sensitive to features of his environment that he would usually ignore. Like the cats in Key's first experiment, the more stimuli around him he has to select from the more disturbing the experience becomes. It is believed that this peculiar sensitizing effect of LSD is due to a specific action of the drug on the brain's filtering mechanisms. The effect is as though the band-width of stimuli allowed to reach consciousness has been enormously increased. This theory helps to explain some of the odd results obtained with LSD in the human experimental laboratory. For example, in Chapter Three we saw how, unlike amphetamine which has a more uniformly arousing effect, LSD markedly lengthens the individual's reaction time despite the fact that physiologically he seems to be more alert. The reason is that because LSD increases the number of irrelevant stimuli affecting the subject he finds it difficult to sort out the particular tone or light to which he is supposed to be responding. Another experiment from Professor Bradley's laboratory has, in fact, demonstrated a similar effect in animals [37]. There measurements were made of the time it took for cats to carry out a simple conditioned response when a light came on. Sometimes the light came on alone, sometimes it was accompanied by a series of brief tones. The effect of LSD on the animal's reaction time depended on whether or not the tones were also present. When the light came on by itself the animal responded more quickly under LSD than after being given a saline injection. However, when the light and tones were presented together reactions under LSD were *slower* than normal, indicating that the animal was being distracted by the additional auditory stimulation.

All of the experiments just described illustrate how the psychopharmacologist tries to relate the brain to behaviour by examining the effect of drugs on the gross physiology or neural circuitry of the brain. If we took a closer look at the nervous system, however, we would see that it is made up of a vast number of nerve cells, or neurones, even a simple brain circuit being an intricate network of such cells. At a more fundamental level psychotropic drugs exert their action on the brain – and hence on behaviour – by altering the electrochemical activity of the neurones themselves and it is here that a good deal of basic research in psychopharmacology is carried out. By miniaturizing electrophysiological recording it has now become possible to monitor the activity of individual nerve cells into which tiny microelectrodes have been inserted. The cell's response to a drug can then be studied in much the same way as when recording from larger areas of brain tissue. The drug itself may be injected in the usual way into the bloodstream and allowed to reach the brain through the normal circulation. Alternatively, a more precise technique may be used, called *iontophoresis*. Here the drug is placed directly in the immediate vicinity of the neurone from which the recording is being taken. This is achieved by combining the recording electrode with a micropipette containing a solution of the drug. A current is passed through the solution, causing the active ion of the drug to migrate through the pipette barrel into the cell membrane. As the drug exerts its effect, a simultaneous recording can then be made of the changes occurring within the cell.

Research on the physiology of nerve cells has suggested that an important site of drug action is probably at the synapses, the junctions where individual neurones meet and influence each other's activity. In reality there is no physical contact between neurones, the synapse actually consisting of a minute space across which 'information' is transmitted from one cell to another. Synaptic transmission is now known to occur through chemical means, neurones influencing their neighbours by secreting tiny quantities of transmitter substances across the gaps between them. A number of chemicals occur naturally in the nervous system and, with varying degrees of certainty, all of them have been considered as possible transmitter substances. Two, acetylcholine and norepinephrine, are definitely known to act in this way; while similar properties have also been ascribed to several others, including 5-hydroxytryptamine or serotonin and gamma-aminobutyric acid, GABA for short.

A significant feature of synaptic connexions which should be mentioned at this point is that some synapses perform an excitatory and others an inhibitory function. It is indeed a general property of the nervous system that wherever one finds mechanisms that increase excitability these are always matched by restraining mechanisms which serve to damp down activity. The necessity of being able to maintain homeostasis in the brain in this way becomes obvious if one tries to visualize what would happen if inhibition did not exist. To paraphrase the comments of one famous neurophysiologist: energy potential within the human skull is such that if inhibition were not there to keep our brains in check, we would all literally blow our tops! The opposition between excitation and inhibition occurs in many forms in the nervous system. We have already seen, for example, how at a different level an elaborate stop-go circuitry in the brain controls even a simple behavioural reaction like the galvanic skin response. At the cellular level excitatory and inhibitory synapses can be distinguished physiologically by the sort of electrical change recorded from neurones and attempts have been made to relate the two kinds of synaptic connexion to particular transmitter substances. Some experts, for example, believe that GABA is an inhibitory transmitter. However, the picture is probably much more complicated than that. For one thing it is known that the transmitter substance, acetylcholine, has both excitatory and inhibitory properties, its effect partly depending on where in the nervous system it is found. Furthermore, it is now thought that whether a synapse is excitatory or inhibitory may depend as much upon the anatomical structure of a neurone's synaptic membrane as upon the transmitter substance secreted from it. Finally, it should be remembered that each nerve cell in the brain may receive many thousands of synaptic contacts. Its activity at any one time will therefore be the result of a complex interaction between innumerable excitatory and inhibitory influences, each involving an elaborate chain of biochemical processes.

These difficulties have naturally not deterred psychopharmacologists from speculating about the way in which drugs affect neuronal activity. In general terms they probably do so by modifying the action of the brain's neurohumours or some chemical precursor or metabolite of the latter. Thus a drug whose chemical structure is similar to that of a transmitter substance may flood synaptic receptor sites and imitate the action of the natural transmitter. Alternatively, drugs of different chemical structure may occupy the receptor sites and block the access of the natural transmitter substance to them. These mimicking or blocking actions may occur at both excitatory and inhibitory synapses so that similar changes in behaviour can result from quite opposite effects on the nerve cells. We can see an example of this if we compare the actions of two drugs, pentetrazol and strychnine, both of which have powerful stimulant effects on behaviour. Pentetrazol appears to produce its effects by mimicking the action of acetylcholine at excitatory synapses. Strychnine, on the other hand, has the same overt effect but here by selectively blockading inhibitory synapses, so allowing excitatory neurones to fire unrestrained.

Another way in which some psychotropic drugs may act is not by interfering with the secretion of the natural neurohumours themselves but with some other part of the biochemical process in which they are involved during neuronal firing. The transmitter substances go through a well-defined metabolic cycle in which they are synthesized, stored and then, after release at the synaptic junction, broken down by a specific antagonist. Each phase in this cycle is vulnerable to the effects of drugs. The purpose of the last, destruction, stage is to prevent the transmitter substance needlessly continuing to act at the synapse after it has done its job; thus incidentally providing another example of how the brain protects itself against disruption. In the case of the two established transmitters, norepinephrine and acetylcholine, the cycle just described is well-understood. Acetylcholine, for example, is broken down by the enzyme cholinesterase and a number of drugs that excite the nervous system do so because they prevent cholinesterase inactivating acetylcholine. One such anticholin-esterase agent is physostigmine, a drug of limited medical use but with a colourful history. Physostigmine is derived from the 'ordeal' bean, so named because it was once used in parts of Africa in trials of witchcraft, the poor victim being forced to eat the bean as a test of his innocence. Often death ensued, following widespread excitation of the central and autonomic nervous systems. Those who survived were pronounced not guilty, though it is thought that they did so because, with the confidence of the innocent, they consumed the bean so rapidly that they were protected by vomiting from its fatal effects.

Apart from these rather drastic behavioural reactions – which incidentally characterize a number of the non-therapeutic drugs used in basic research of the kind just described – how far is it possible to relate the action of drugs on nerve cells to more subtle psychological processes? No final answer can yet be given to that question, though an area in which there has been considerable speculation is in trying to explain the biochemical basis of abnormal mental states, particularly schizophrenia. All of the theories proposed make use of the general notion that schizophrenia is due to an excess, a deficiency, or some more complex imbalance of the brain's neurohumours. Two kinds of evidence have been used to support such theories. One arises from the fact that a number of hallucinogenic drugs are of similar chemical structure to some of the substances that occur naturally in the brain. Thus, LSD is chemically very similar to serotonin, and mescaline similar to norepinephrine. The second source of evidence concerns the anatomical distribution of the brain's neurohumours. For example, high concentrations of serotonin are found in the hypothalamus and in other subcortical areas that control emotional expression, an aspect of behaviour that is of course grossly disturbed in schizophrenia.

Unfortunately, none of these theories of schizophrenia has so far been entirely substantiated by experimental facts, and solution to the problem in terms of brain biochemistry is little nearer than it ever was. This is not surprising when it is realized that even taking the intermediate step of relating one level of brain function to another is itself fraught with many difficulties. Take, for instance, the effect of an established drug like amphetamine on the apparently simple processes of central nervous excitation and inhibition. Microelectrode recordings have shown that, when applied locally to the brain by iontophoresis, amphetamine has a mainly inhibitory action on the electrical activity of individual neurones in the brainstem. Yet, as we saw earlier, its effect on the brain as a whole is to increase excitability. That example illustrates just one of the many gaps in our knowledge both about drug effects and about brain function. The field of research from which it happens to be taken forms, too, only one of a wide range of sciences concerned with the biology of behaviour. The spectrum of interests represented varies from the nature of synaptic transmission, through the functional significance of the brain's circuitry, to the causes of unpredictable behaviour in female socialites. Scientists who stand at different points along this continuum can, with varying degrees of certainty, make use of facts obtained by their neighbours. Those who occupy its opposite extremes can scarcely communicate sensibly with each other at the present time and it may be many decades, or even centuries, before the psychologist and the biochemist can even begin to translate the other's terminology into his own. I think we can be certain, however, that progress towards that end will be hastened by an increasing contribution from psychopharmacology, which provides a logical testing-ground for theories wishing to chase the mind to its place within the nerve cell.

Drugs in Daily Life 9

The day before I started to write this chapter the Ministry of Health published its annual report for 1967. The picture the report paints of the British population is of a depressed, anxiety-ridden, and sleepless community rattling on the doors of its general practitioners and psychiatric outpatient clinics seeking relief for its mental suffering. During the year in question British doctors responded to the call for help by putting pen to prescription-pad forty million times. More than three-quarters of these Government-stamped passports to lotus-land were exchanged for sleeping pills or tranquillizers and the remainder for mood-elevating drugs. Not content in its quest for equanimity, the drug-hungry British public also prescribed for itself vast quantities of other remedies for its psychological malaise. The most potent of these was bought daily over the counters of the local bars. Others were chemically inactive or at least medicinally irrelevant, though probably as psychologically therapeutic as some of those obtained officially through the National Health

Service. Whether we like it or not – and we appear to like it very much – drugs are intruding more and more into our daily lives. The demand for drugs ranges from the request by the ordinary citizen for a bottle of nerve calmers to see him through a temporary crisis to the physiological craving of the addict caught in a vicious circle of elation and despair that leads frequently to personal degradation and sometimes to death.

Several factors have been held responsible for this drug explosion in society. A commonly quoted cause is the increased anxiety associated with the stress of modern living. By itself this explanation is certainly too facile. In earlier times of less affluence and social security the stress must have been greater and the level of anxiety in the community much higher than they are now. Indeed, as will be argued later, there are good reasons for believing that some forms of drug-taking can be put down to quite the opposite cause, to the search for ways of relieving boredom in a world in which most biological and economic needs are satiated. Other villains who have been blamed are the pharmaceutical companies, for their commercialism and lavish advertising, and the medical profession, for its overenthusiastic prescribing of drugs. In the case of the drug companies the criticism is certainly justified to some extent. At the same time it should be remembered that one of the most mentally disruptive and addictive drugs to which the public is exposed, namely alcohol, does not even originate from them. Yet, because of the undoubted pleasures and despite the dangers associated with it, alcohol enjoys relatively unrestricted advertising and distribution with the full approval of society. As for the medical profession, it must of course carry immediate responsibility for the massive administration of officially recognized psychotropic drugs. In its defence, however, some of the difficulties under which it works must be borne in mind. It is now widely accepted that a large proportion – perhaps as high as eighty per cent – of patients seeking help from their general practitioners have some sort of psychological difficulty. Theoretically such people might be best treated by simple psychotherapy or counselling. For the over-worked GP this is out of the question. Even in the busy specialist clinic it may not always be feasible. Doctors are hardly to be blamed, therefore, if they have recourse to drugs which, as they themselves admit, may often have only palliative effects. The situation is not helped by a drug-sophisticated public which is sometimes aware of, and ready to demand, the latest remedies before the doctor himself has become fully acquainted with them. Even if he had time personally to weigh up the evidence for and against a new drug, the doctor would find himself bewildered by the contradictory findings of numerous clinical trials. For let us not deceive ourselves. While the *safety* of new drugs is now taken care of extremely well, the *efficacy* of many of them is by no means well-established. In the case of some, this may be because they are of no value anyway. In other cases it may simply be difficult to decide, either because different trials of a drug have been carried out under conditions that are not entirely comparable, or because the issue is befogged by some trials that add nothing to our knowledge, though a good deal to the weight of our scientific journals.

All of us, then, from the unhappy consumer to the research psychopharmacologist – and not forgetting the writer of popular books on the subject – must share responsibility for the current interest in drugs. Of course, not all of this interest is morbid nor, in most cases, do drugs bring anything but benefit to the individual taking them – even if they sometimes do so by acting merely as placebos. But if drugs are to figure even larger in our lives – and there is every reason to believe that they will – it is desirable that society should be aware of the facts and fallacies underlying their use. That, to some extent, is the *raison d'être* for books of this kind. It is also why this particular book has so far been written from a fairly strict scientific viewpoint and illustrated wherever possible by experimental evidence, which I trust has not been too indigestible. The story would not be complete, however, unless we were prepared to shut the doors of the laboratory and see whether what we have learned there can help us to understand some of the uses to which drugs are put in daily life and some of the problems that they pose for society at large.

Let us look, first, at the legitimate outlet for most psychotropic drugs, their use in the treatment of the psychiatric patient. Faced with a national bill for drugs that rises annually, many must wonder whether a corresponding improvement in the mental health of the community has occurred. A cynic might well reach the opposite conclusion, for desire is all too often the slave of its own satisfaction. Such cynicism should not blind us to the undoubted relief that drugs have brought to many mentally ill people, though an important point about their use in psychiatric treatment should also be borne in mind. In most cases psychotropic drugs are not curative in the same way in which, say, antibiotics are in the treatment of physical diseases caused by viruses. This is because most psychiatric disorders are not diseases in the strict medical sense. Instead, they are more in the nature of disturbed patterns of behaviour and are therefore subject to many social and psychological influences. Whether a patient improves or not may depend as much on the changes that are occurring within himself or in his environment as upon the chemical action of the drug he is taking. Sometimes, especially in neurotic conditions, the passage of time alone may help to heal. Take the case of a man suffering from depression which is reactive to some financial crisis. A favourable swing in his fortunes on the Stock Exchange will certainly relieve his gloom, though a bottle of antidepressives and a word of encouragement from the psychiatrist may help meantime to see him through his difficulties. Often, however, it is necessary to combine the use of drugs with a more deliberate attempt to remove the patient's symptoms. This might take the form of intensive psychotherapy or one of the newer methods based on learning principles [3]. The theory behind these 'behaviour therapy' techniques, as they are called, is that neurotic symptoms are conditioned habits which can be removed by getting the patient to unlearn them. When a drug is used in conjunction with such methods it is chosen so that it will alter the patient's physiological state in a predictable way and so speed up the deconditioning or extinction process. The drugs that do this are the depressants, such as sedatives and tranquillizers. A couple of examples will help to illustrate the logic of using drugs in this way to treat neurotic symptoms.

Consider, first of all, the case of a patient with an intractable tic, such as the irresistible urge to shake his head every few minutes. The hypothesis to explain the symptom would be that it developed originally as a way of relieving anxiety, though now it may serve no purpose at all. Indeed, it is more likely to *cause* the patient anxiety and embarrassment. A method of eliminating the tic would be to get the patient to practise it intensively. Under these conditions of 'massed practice' a certain amount of inhibition will build up in the nervous system; or, to put it in everyday language, the patient will weary of performing his unwanted habit. Eventually he will start taking rests from it, the same rest pauses or 'blocks' which, as we saw earlier in the book, occur on all monotonous tasks. After several sessions of practice the rest pauses will gradually become longer and more frequent until eventually the patient will be taking more time off from the tic than that spent performing it. Finally the habit will die out completely. Now, we know from laboratory research that depressant drugs increase the proneness to inhibition and hence the tendency to take rest pauses. The effectiveness of this 'negative practice' technique, as it is called, will therefore be much enhanced if we give the patient a small dose of sedative during his treatment.

In the example just described the drug will have helped to eliminate the neurotic habit by affecting the extinction process directly. The second case to be mentioned is rather different. Here the drug acts indirectly by reducing anxiety in people undergoing deconditioning for symptoms of a phobic nature. The patient may complain of an uncontrollable fear of particular situations or objects, such as cats, trains, or wide open spaces. If the symptom is treated by behaviour therapy the patient will be put through a course of what is called 'progressive desensitization'. As the name implies, this involves exposing the person to the phobic object very gradually until he is able to face it with equanimity. Supposing the patient is afraid of large black dogs. Treatment might start in one of several ways. The patient might be shown a large black dog at a distance, sufficiently far away for it to be only mildly alarming. Alternatively, he might be encouraged to fondle a small black dog or even just look at pictures of dogs. Whichever method is used, the patient must be made fully at ease before he is exposed to dogs that are physically nearer to him or more like his original phobic object. At each stage in treatment the patient is calmed down by verbal reassurance though, if anxiety is very high, tranquillizing drugs may be required as well. If drugs are used the dose is gradually tailed off as the patient begins to lose his phobia. This is done in order to prevent him becoming too dependent on them as a permanent solution to his anxiety.

Of course, in neither of these two cases is the use of drugs essential to treatment and many behaviour therapists prefer to rely on purely psychological techniques to cure patients of the kind described. There are, however, other forms of behaviour therapy in which drugs are an integral part of the treatment procedure. These belong to the category of 'aversion therapies', so called because they are used in an attempt to eliminate patterns of behaviour that are socially undesirable or distressing to those around the patient – though not necessarily to the patient himself. Such disorders include alcoholism, compulsive gambling, and various sexual perversions, such as fetishism and transvestism. The principle behind the aversion therapies is that the habit to be eliminated is repeatedly associated with some unpleasant stimulus. The theory is that the patient will eventually avoid performing the habit, say drinking alcohol, because through conditioning the sight and smell of his favourite beverage will excite in him feelings of repugnance rather than pleasure. Almost anything distasteful to the patient could be used as the punishing stimulus, but if a drug is chosen it is usually one that produces physical sensations of nausea. One such drug is apomorphine which has often been used in aversion therapy, particularly with alcoholics.

Compared with other types of behaviour therapy, such as progressive desensitization, the aversion methods have not been particularly successful. There are several reasons for this. Some, probably of rather minor importance, are purely technical and arise from defects in the treatment procedure itself. One concerns the timing of the associations between the response being punished and the aversive stimulus. Experiments on conditioning have established that the interval between these two events, and the order in which they occur, is crucial if proper learning is to take place. In the case of drug-induced aversion exact timing may be impossible to arrange. Even if the drug is administered by injection, the onset of nausea will not be easy to predict and in any case it will vary widely from one individual to the next. Another problem is that apomorphine may itself have a centrally depressant effect which will, of course, actually slow down the very learning that the therapist is trying to achieve. Incidentally, a similar difficulty can arise in the treatment of alcoholism anyway, because the depressant action of the alcoholic drink to which the patient is being averted will also interfere with conditioning; though this is easily solved by getting him simply to taste the alcohol and then to spit it out after each learning trial.

In order to overcome the other two problems, behaviour therapists have tried alternatives to apomorphine as the aversive stimulus. The most common of these is electric shock, which has the advantage that the timing and intensity of the punishment can be controlled much more precisely. Unfortunately, none of the modifications to the techniques of aversion therapy has improved much upon its effectiveness and the real reasons for its modest success rate probably go much deeper. They almost certainly have something to do with the nature of the disorders in which aversion therapy is normally used. The alcoholic, for example, is not just someone with a drinking problem. The basic defect from which he suffers infiltrates his whole physical and mental existence so that many medical and social agencies have to be mobilized to deal with the chaos that alcoholism leaves in its wake. Compulsive gambling is scarcely less intractable. The gambler is frequently a heavy drinker, if not an alcoholic, as well. He is a risk-taker not only on the pin-tables and in the betting shop but in everything he does, living his life with a disastrously small margin of error. Family and business relationships are disrupted so much that, like the alcoholic, no one person – and certainly no drug – can hope to rescue the gambler from the roundabout of debt on which he inevitably finds himself. Another important feature of all of the conditions to which aversion therapy is applied is that there is a strong element of pleasure in them. Unlike the anxiety neurotic, whose symptoms are agony to him, the alcoholic, the compulsive gambler, and the sexual pervert all enjoy what they do. Admittedly they may subsequently feel guilty about their fall from grace, but this is usually too far removed in time to have much effect and the habit will tend to be maintained by the powerful reinforcing influence of immediate gratification. Taking all of these factors into account, it is not surprising that present aversion methods, whether using drugs or not, have had only limited success.

In practice very few neurotic patients are treated by the strict behaviour therapy methods just described. This is partly because there are not many patients who have a simple tic or an isolated phobia. Most have complex psychological difficulties that are not amenable to any of the behaviour therapy techniques so far devised. Traditionally, of course, the psychiatrist has dealt with this sort of patient by letting him talk out his problems. Even this is a kind of informal behaviour therapy in that the psychiatrist tries by verbal persuasion to 'decondition' the patient out of his irrational fears. As with behaviour therapy proper, drugs may be used to control the physiological aspects of the patient's anxiety, thus providing the psychiatrist with a simple way of breaking into the vicious circle that often perpetuates neurotic symptoms. Of course, there is nothing very original or scientific about this form of treatment. Psychiatrists have been treating their patients like that for years. The main difference is that, for good or ill, the doctor now has a much wider range of psychotropic drugs to choose from. All of these are claimed by their makers to have some special anti-anxiety or antidepressive property not shared by any other drug. Actually, as far as the minor tranquillizers are concerned, it is doubtful whether dose for dose they are any more effective than the older sedatives. However, compared with the drugs they have tended to replace, namely the barbiturates, they do have two advantages. One is that the risk of death from overdosage is slighter. The other is that they are rather less addictive though the risk of psychological dependence on them is by no means absent. As for antidepressive drugs, their special contribution to the treatment of neurosis is even more dubious. Chronically anxious people are often depressed as well and may be treated accordingly with antidepressives. Some experts believe, however, that when used in this way such drugs are acting merely as tranquillizers and are not specifically antidepressive at all. This idea fits in with the research findings described in Chapter Seven, namely that the physiological make-up of patients with neurotic or reactive depression is really no different from that of other dysthymic individuals. They could be, and sometimes are, treated just as effectively with sedative or tranquillizing drugs.

If drug treatment of neurotic symptoms is not as sophisticated as the pharmaceutical companies would sometimes have us believe, this is surely not true of more severe mental illness. Or is it? Only a fool would deny the place of antidepressive drugs in the relief of some forms of profound depression, though it is interesting to note that even now one of the most successful treatments for this condition is non-pharmacological, namely electroconvulsive therapy. The most loudly applauded contribution of drugs to psychiatric care, however, is in the treatment of schizo-phrenia and the beginning of the 'modern drug era' in psychiatry is usually dated from the introduction of chlorpromazine. There is no doubt that this major tranquillizer and its derivatives have helped to bring under control crippling psychotic symptoms that would otherwise require intensive hospital custody. Now the schizophrenic patient stays a shorter time in hospital and is protected to some extent from the additional handicap of institutional neurosis, the insidious canker of social and emo-tional deterioration that follows prolonged hospitalization.

Although some of these changes can be put down to drug therapy, it should also be remembered that the advent of the major tranquillizers coincided with the beginning of an attitude towards mental illness which is in general more liberal and humanitarian. This has resulted in a shift, over the past twenty years, in the pattern of psychiatric treatment. Though slow to die completely, the image of the asylum-incarcerated lunatic is gradually disappearing as more and more patients are cared for in acute admission units, many of which are attached to general hospitals, and then later rehabilitated in the community. Social, occupational and physical methods may all be combined into what has sometimes been called 'total push' therapy, which tries to keep the schizophrenic functioning at a level that is not too unacceptable to those around him. The main role of drugs in this programme of therapy is that they make the patient more accessible to human contact, so enabling other, non-physical, forms of treatment to be put into effect. In principle, therefore, the part played by drugs is similar to that which they play in the treatment of neurosis, though there are some differences. For one thing, the behaviour that needs correcting is much more deranged, as well as being both less understandable and less understood. The contribution to treatment made by a drug's chemical action is also much more decisive, though it is doubtful whether drugs given by themselves would materially alter the outcome of schizophrenia. In fact, treatment of the condition with tranquillizers is largely ineffective unless they are used in conjunction with an active programme of social and industrial rehabilitation. It is a combination of both forms of treatment, rather than either alone, that seems to work best.

In no sense, therefore, can we yet talk of a chemical cure for schizophrenia. Shall we ever be able to do so? That depends very much on what schizophrenia eventually turns out to be. At the present time opinion is by no means unanimous. Those who cling to an orthodox medical viewpoint regard schizophrenia as a distinct disease or group of diseases determined to a large extent by heredity. The term 'disease' is used here in the strict medical sense that those with a particular condition are somehow qualitatively different from those without it. People who hold this view look forward to the day when some future Nobel Prize winner will discover the discrete biochemical disorder that is responsible for the disease. At the opposite extreme are some who regard schizophrenia quite differently. They consider it to be a failure in interpersonal relationships, somewhat akin to a neurotic breakdown, and seek the cause in the patient's family background. Such people tend to play down the genetic evidence and look upon biochemical theories as little more than red herrings.

There is also a third opinion that is something of a compromise between the other two and, on the whole, more consistent with the known facts about schizophrenia. That is that in most, though not necessarily all, cases the schizophrenic reaction is nothing more than an extreme variant of normal brain function. We have already seen how individual differences in personality are related to variations in brain activity. Schizophrenia, or rather the different forms of schizophrenia, may simply represent extremes of some of the personality types found among the general population. Several different kinds of evidence would support this view. The so-called schizoid personality has long been recognized as someone who shows many of the abortive features of the schizophrenic patient, but who never actually has a psychiatric breakdown. Furthermore, some of the individual symptoms of schizophrenia, such as odd thoughts and perceptions, occur transiently in otherwise perfectly normal people. Other evidence comes from the parallel that is often drawn between schizophrenic thinking and the way highly creative people think. Many astute observers of human nature have made this comparison, notably John Dryden in his famous words:

> Great wits are sure to madness near alli'd
> And thin partitions do their bounds divide.

Formal psychological studies of individual differences in cognitive 'style' have now actually shown that the loose thinking characteristic of creativity is not unlike that found in the schizophrenic and probably has a similar neurophysiological basis. In fact, one genetic theory of psychosis has seriously proposed that schizophrenia is the biological penalty man must pay for the evolution of flexible, creative thought.

This 'normal variant' view of schizophrenia differs, therefore, in a number of ways from the other two theories mentioned earlier. Like the disease theory it takes account of biochemical and genetic factors, though it puts slightly different emphasis on them. Of course, all behaviour has biochemical correlates but their significance for the understanding of schizophrenia may be nothing more than that of providing another biological level at which we can describe the condition, just as we can describe anxiety in biochemical terms. If such factors take on greater relevance than that it may be because drugs used to modify the schizophrenic's behaviour – or anybody else's for that matter – act ultimately on the biochemistry of the brain. As for genetic factors, it certainly looks as though the tendency to have a schizophrenic breakdown is strongly determined by heredity. But then so are many other human characteristics, such as intelligence, extraversion, proneness to anxiety, and so on. Some people believe that, like these normal traits, the predisposition to schizophrenia is present in everyone; or, as one of my psychiatric colleagues once jovially put it, 'all of us have a touch of the schizophrenias'. Whether the tendency comes out in the form of a psychiatric breakdown may depend on many factors: the number of 'schizophrenic genes' present, the strength or weakness of other genetically determined personality traits, the cultural norms against which the person is judged, and, as the psychological theorists point out, the individual's remote and immediate life experiences.

From what has been said is it possible to predict how schizophrenia will be treated in the future? If the disease theory were to prove correct then treatment would be fairly simple, at least in principle. Once the biochemical dysfunction had been found, discovering a method of reversing it could not be far behind. A drug would have to be synthesized which would turn the chemical lock that some believe to be permanently jammed – or too freely opened – in the schizophrenic brain. Should purely psychological theories prevail, the future role of drugs might be a relatively minor one, as social scientists discover new ways of preventing or modifying the pathological family patterns that are said to occur in schizophrenia. The third possibility, that schizophrenia will only be understandable in terms of normal brain function, presents a bleak prospect, certainly not the dramatic solution within the decade forecast by some optimists. If, as I suspect, this is the most likely alternative, we shall have to be content to let basic research in all the behavioural sciences grind on its way towards a greater knowledge of how the normal brain works. Progress there will certainly be supplemented by the discovery of new drugs which are more selective in their effects than any available at the present time. These will enable the psychiatrist to bring each aspect of mental activity under precise chemical control. If any particular psychological function is disordered, then administering the appropriate drug in the correct dose will shift the corresponding brain system just the right amount towards normality.

To see how the treatment of schizophrenia might benefit from these advances in psychopharmacology, let us look at the following example. Supposing we wish to cure a paranoid patient of a persecutory delusion that his neighbours are broadcasting obscene stories about him through the cathode ray tube of his television set. It is thought that bizarre beliefs of this kind arise because of the defective filtering of information that occurs in psychotic states. As we saw earlier, the band-width of the brain's filter can sometimes get broader than it should be; then the individual begins to pay attention to stimuli and events around him that he would usually ignore. The intrusion of odd irrelevant thoughts occurs momentarily in all of us from time to time, but we quickly suppress them as of no account. The schizophrenic is unable to do so and the events may begin to take on significance for him. Eventually he may build up an elaborate delusional system around them which has no basis in reality. Now at some time in the future it may be possible to develop a drug which will damp down the precise brain mechanisms responsible for delusions developing. Drugs of a different kind, but with an equally narrow spectrum of action, will be used to control other disorders of brain function found in schizophrenia, such as hallucinations and incongruous emotional reactions. At the moment all of these symptoms are controlled reasonably well by chlorpromazine and other phenothiazine drugs. In the future such 'blunderbuss' drugs will probably be replaced by a whole range of psychotropic agents each having a very specialized action on the brain.

Of course, it is quite possible that all three theories of schizophrenia I mentioned will prove to be correct. It is quite common in medicine to find that the same group of symptoms arise for a variety of reasons. Take a simple example, that of mild disturbance of the thyroid gland. A person with this defect may show profuse sweating, rapid pulse, and other signs of jitteriness. Superficially he may be hard to distinguish from someone who is just basically a very anxious personality. Yet the cause, and the remedy, are different. Similarly, in the case of schizophrenia one rare form, periodic catatonia, is already known to be associated with a disturbance of the body's metabolism of nitrogen. Schizophrenic behaviour can also occur in the presence of damage to certain areas of the brain, especially the temporal lobes. Future treatment of schizophrenia is therefore likely to include many different techniques: chemical, surgical and behavioural. In practice, more than one method will probably be used together in the same patient, just as happens at present. Consider again the paranoid patient I mentioned a moment ago. In addition to having his defective filtering system controlled with drugs, such a patient might undergo psychological retraining to modify any existing behaviour which the brain abnormality had caused, such as avoidance of situations associated with his delusion. For this purpose it should be possible to devise suitable behaviour therapy techniques of the kind described earlier. These have already been applied on a small scale to psychotic behaviour and together with suitable drugs they might eventually make a valuable contribution to the future treatment of schizophrenic patients.

Naturally, in order to use drugs in a rational way in psychiatric treatment, we need to know much more than we do at present about the physiological basis of personality and its abnormalities. This does not just apply to schizophrenia, but is true of all mental illness. Even in conditions less complicated than schizophrenia many quite fundamental questions remain unanswered. Consequently, to the outsider, drug treatment in psychiatry still looks a rather hit-or-miss affair. Actually it is not quite as bad as it seems because, through a combination of trial and error and accumulated clinical experience, psychiatry has developed a series of rules of thumb for treating patients with drugs. In practice, these work quite well, but psychotropic drugs could be used even more effectively if the psychiatrist had at his disposal more objective indicators of their effects. There are really two problems here. One is to select the right drug in the first place. The other is, having decided, to ensure that the drug is given in the optimum dose for the particular patient being treated. Typical of the first problem is the difficulty of deciding whether a patient is suffering from a neurotic or a psychotic form of depression. The second problem is typically that of fixing the right amount of sedative to give an anxious patient and of measuring its effects as treatment proceeds. In Chapter Seven we saw some of the ways in which basic research is trying to answer these questions. As yet, few of the techniques described there have passed over into clinical practice, but this will inevitably happen as psychiatric diagnosis becomes more scientific. Eventually, before he is treated, each patient will be put through a battery of psycho-physiological tests to decide which drug and how much of it he requires. Further tests at intervals throughout treatment will enable the effects of the drug to be monitored quite precisely. This matching of the patient to his treatment will form an integral part of the psychiatry of the future, though it may be many decades before such a situation is fully realized. At present the rate at which new drugs are discovered far outstrips our under-standing of the conditions they are intended to cure, and one of psychiatry's most urgent problems is to catch up on the progress that is being made in the basic science of pharma-cology.

With this brief glimpse into the future of psychiatric treatment let us turn to a question of more immediate concern. So far in this chapter I have implicitly assumed that the use of drugs to correct mental disharmony is always a good thing, if done under the guise of psychiatric treatment. Is this necessarily so? As far as incapacitating mental illness is concerned, either psychotic or neurotic, the answer is not in doubt. But patients with such severe disorders as these form only the core of a much larger group of people suffering from a hotchpotch of relatively minor psychological complaints. This group of mildly unhappy people is a changing one, in that at some time or another it could include any one of us. Its permanent members, however, are chronic hypochondriacs with vague but notoriously intractable physical symptoms, individuals with ill-defined neurotic fears, and many others trying to escape the chores of living, either from boredom or from anxiety. The doctor, often a general practitioner, who prescribes antidepressives or tranquillizers for such people frequently does so fully realizing that they are probably no more weary or worried than he is. The motives that take them to his surgery are many and varied. Some may have genuine psychological problems of which they are unaware or unable to face. In these cases drugs provide only a temporary, and therefore unsatisfactory, solution to their difficulties. Others seeking relief from drugs do so out of the mistaken, but in our society prevalent, notion that any kind of anxiety is a bad thing. This is constantly brought home to us as articles and advertisements in the press and the sight of mindlessly relaxed TV personalities remind us daily of the dangers of nervous tension. Yet in the moderate degree that most people feel it, even under stress, anxiety is a normal biological drive which motivates a good deal of human endeavour. (Without it, I can assure the reader, this book would have progressed little further than a pile of illegible notes!)

Of course, as laboratory studies have quite clearly shown, once anxiety increases beyond a certain optimum level, it does begin to impair psychological efficiency and here tranquillizing drugs are of genuine help in reducing anxiety that is pathologically high. But it is doubtful whether most people experience such excessive anxiety on more than a few occasions in their lives. In fact, the 'worries' that take some people to their doctors with requests for tranquillizers probably derive, not from anxiety at all, but from its opposite – boredom. For, just as a very high level of anxiety is distressing, so also is the feeling of being too un-aroused. As I described in the previous chapter, the brain requires a constant influx of signals to maintain its alertness. At a psychological level this is reflected in what has been described as 'stimulus hunger' or, more pithily, as the need for 'arousal jag'. This desire for stimulation is what motivates the gambler, the sports car driver, the fairground enthusiast, and the house-bound housewife bitching at her husband that he never takes her out any more. Some people, notably rather extraverted individuals, appear to require more frequent and more intense arousal jags than others; while a few seem to have an extraordinary resistance to monotony.

The need for stimulation will increase in most of us, however, if all our desires are satisfied and there is little left to excite us. Since in societies such as ours there are few drives that remain unsatisfied for very long, novel amusements for our hungry minds have constantly to be devised. If these fail or for some reason are unavailable, the less imaginative or more neurotic among us turn in upon their own thoughts and problems and finally take their 'anxieties' to the doctor. He may astutely decide that the trouble is not anxiety at all, but melancholy, and prescribe antidepressive drugs. As it happens these probably will have a stimulating action on the brain but their medicinal effects may be less than the 'change of air' the doctor's elder partner might have prescribed.

Of course, not all of the people I have just described will seek medical help. Some will treat themselves, a practice that is growing as rapidly as the official prescription of drugs in the National Health Service. According to a recent report by the Office of Health Economics, in 1966 the British public treated itself at a cost of seventy-nine million pounds, a sum which was over one-third of the total expenditure on medicines in the United Kingdom for that year [73]. What is it that sends people scurrying to the chemist rather than (or as well as) visiting the GP's surgery? Often it is a minor accident or trivial physical complaint, though psychological factors probably also play a disproportionately large role, both directly and indirectly. Many people with vaguely psychiatric symptoms prefer to treat themselves, as do others with so-called psychosomatic complaints such as skin disorders. The remedies they choose to buy range from relatively powerful drugs like aspirin and codeine to harmless 'placebo' preparations such as vitamins, tonics, and other pick-me-ups. The authors of the report just referred to conclude that on the whole the practice of self-prescription is not detrimental to the nation's health; rather it is complementary to the treatments received through normal medical channels.

While these conclusions are probably true for the majority of the population there is another kind of self-treatment which is much more drastic. That is the tendency for some people to try and solve their psychological problems by having recourse to massive quantities of drugs on which they become partly or totally dependent. Far from solving their difficulties, such people throw a large burden on the psychiatric services because of the social problems that drug addiction itself creates. The drug that is the greatest offender, numerically speaking, is alcohol, but no one needs to be reminded of the increasing scale on which abuse of other drugs is occurring. Alcoholism and other kinds of drug addiction have usually been studied and discussed as separate issues, mainly for historical reasons. Drinking alcohol forms an intrinsic part of the recreational life of Western cultures and society is therefore very tolerant of any deviant behaviour associated with abuse of the drug. It takes a much more censorious attitude towards other drugs such as marihuana, which in fact is probably less dangerous than alcohol and which, among some subcultures in the community, is replacing alcohol as the social drug of choice.

The term 'drug addiction' used in the narrow sense to exclude alcohol, has traditionally been taken to cover drugs which are not socially approved of, except for medical purposes. It has been particularly associated with the abuse of so-called 'hard' drugs, which include the opiates, morphine and heroin, cocaine and various synthetic narcotic analgesics such as pethidine. In addition a number of other drugs are also considered to be potentially habit-forming. These are particularly the barbiturates and amphetamines, but also included are cannabis (marihuana) and some drugs of the hallucinogenic type. Logically there is no reason to separate alcoholism from these other forms of drug addiction, and, in a recent report, the WHO Expert Committee on Mental Health agreed that both should be considered together as basically similar social and psychological problems [76].

Earlier, in 1964, the WHO had recommended that the term 'drug dependence' should replace those of 'drug addiction' and 'drug habituation' [75]. By doing so they took account of the fact that the only property common to all of the drugs under discussion was that 'they are capable of creating a state of mind in certain individuals which is termed psychic dependence'. This state was defined as a 'psychic drive which requires periodic or chronic administration of the drug for pleasure or to avoid discomfort'. Broadening the definition of drug abuse in this way, does, of course, create certain difficulties. Where, for example, does drug dependence begin and end? A recent report on drug addiction by the Office of Health Economics commented as follows [19]:

Some individuals may derive a satisfying or pleasurable sensation from a wide variety of substances taken into the body (e.g. nutmeg, banana-skins, glue-sniffing, snuff, tobacco, alcohol and even food) and continue taking them possibly to an excessive and detrimental degree. Does glue then become a drug of addiction?

The concept of 'drug dependence' does, however, have an important advantage. It recognizes that no clear distinction can be made between different degrees of reliance on drugs as chemical props. The psychological need for tranquillizers of the chronic neurotic shades imperceptibly into the irresistible urge for alcohol of the heavy drinker and this in turn into the delirious craving of the heroin addict. Of course, the pharmacological properties of the drug itself will to some extent determine how dependent on it the individual becomes. Some drugs, particularly those of the 'hard' type, physically grip their victims more intensely and more rapidly than others. However, as a *social* problem in a particular community the chemical addictiveness of a drug may be its least important feature. LSD, for example, is not particularly, if at all, addictive in the strict sense, but a single dose can be mentally very disruptive and its widespread use could be extremely dangerous. Similarly, in our society alcoholism is a considerable threat to the health of the community as a whole simply by virtue of the sheer number of people dependent on alcohol compared with any other drug.

It is being increasingly realized, then, that progress in the understanding and control of drug dependence will come, less from labelling this or that drug as addictive or non-addictive, but more from trying to delineate the precise factors that determine why a given individual becomes dependent on a particular drug. What are these factors? One of obvious importance is availability. In a broad sense this is determined by how far a community accepts a drug as socially harmless or not. Thus, opium smoking is endemic in China but banned in Britain. Here, on the other hand, undue dependence on alcohol is said to involve over 300,000 people, 70,000 of whom are obvious and chronic alcoholics. By comparison, narcotic addicts are relatively uncommon, the number known to the Home Office in 1966 being about 1,300. While this is certainly an underestimate, it is interesting to note that around the same time the figure for heroin addiction in Hong Kong alone was nearly 11,000, a rate for the population which is one hundred times that of Great Britain [19]. For the individual, of course, availability will be largely a function of immediate supply and demand, despite the attitudes that prevail in society generally. Even where the community imposes rigid controls over drugs it declares to be harmful, illicit means will be found to supply such drugs to those who wish to take them. This may range from breaking into the local chemist's shop to highly organized international smuggling rings for distributing narcotic drugs.

Given the availability of drugs in the community, an important factor which will decide the pattern of addiction will be the extent of exposure to different drugs. In the case of alcohol few of us escape; indeed those who do are looked upon as socially 'switched off'. Conditioning to alcohol starts imperceptibly and proceeds without comment from others. Sometimes it may begin at a very early age. In the city in which I am writing it is not unknown for quite young children to be discovered 'under the influence', having been initiated into the delights of alcohol by their inebriated parents. Partly as a result of this, Glasgow has the worst record for alcoholism in the country. An incredibly high proportion of its inhabitants stagger drunkenly through their daily lives, while at least a quarter of the patients admitted to its psychiatric hospitals have alcoholism as a primary or contributory factor in their illnesses. Compared with alcohol, exposure to other drugs is harder to come by, though if one can judge from the figures for dependence this is scarcely true of medically useful drugs such as amphetamines and barbiturates. One estimate of the number of drug misusers in the United Kingdom in 1966 suggested that 80,000 people had some dependence on amphetamines, while the figure for barbiturates was even higher, probably being nearer 100,000. It was also estimated that, in addition to those dependent on prescribed amphetamines, a further 80,000 were using these drugs illicitly. In the same year the illicit use of cannabis was thought to involve 24,000 people [19].

It is this illicit use of drugs which has been identified as the core of the nation's drug problem since, if left uncontrolled, there is a danger of spreading exposure to potentially addictive drugs. Thus, although the absolute incidence of narcotic addiction is low in Great Britain, its rate of increase is alarmingly high, the number of addicts doubling every one-and-a-half years. The situation is particularly serious since the increase involves mainly young people. In 1959 there were no recorded heroin addicts under the age of 20, but by 1966 there were 317. The spread of addiction is largely due to existing addicts 'infecting' others who come into contact with them, most new addicts acquiring the habit from those already dependent on drugs. This does not mean that exposure to drugs inevitably leads even to mild dependence on them. Often the experience may consist of nothing more than casual 'pot-smoking' sessions indulged in by rebellious adolescents. If the drugs they take come in the form of pills they may even be vague about what these contain and in many cases will be driven more by the illegality of what they are doing or by the desire to conform with their group than by any pleasure they obtain from the drug itself. It has been argued, however, that even this form of drug-taking has inherent dangers because it may lead the individual to try out 'harder' drugs. The evidence on which this assumption is based is that almost all heroin addicts, for example, have graduated to narcotics from other drugs like amphetamines and cannabis. The risk is probably a social rather than a pharmacological one, for there is no reason to suppose that experience of one drug increases the physical desire to take another. What is more likely is that, once having made contact with the drug-taking subcultures in society, the individual finds himself increasingly caught up in their web and tempted to seek the new excitement of more powerfully addictive drugs.

Availability of drugs and exposure to them together provide the social background against which individual dependency develops. But why is it that some people either never experience the desire for drugs or feel free to take them or leave them as they wish, while others cannot live without them? Of all the questions that are asked about drug dependence this is one of the most difficult to answer. In reply we can make profound, though not always helpful, statements that such people suffer from personality disorders which make them incapable of resisting the tempting pleasures afforded by drugs. Those who are not psychologists might rephrase this and say simply that they are weak-willed and lacking in moral fibre. In fact, the immediate causes of drug dependency are multiple. Those that operate in one situation may not do so in another, the exact cause varying according to the context in which a particular form of drug dependency arises. In some cases the reason may have to be sought in the individual's social environment. For example, the high rate of alcoholism in Glasgow certainly derives in part, though not entirely, from the appalling conditions under which many people live. It is not surprising that some try to escape from the squalor of their surroundings into the oblivion of alcoholic intoxication.

Here solving the problem is a difficult and gradual process. While much may be done – as in this case it is – to improve the physical environment by providing better housing and other facilities, the traditions of the past set a pattern of drinking behaviour which is much harder to eradicate. Sometimes the individual may seek the solace of drugs for personal reasons. Many a man has been driven to drink and many a woman to the drug cupboard because of an intolerable home situation which, if it persists, may lead to chronic dependence. Among the young, the affluent and the bored the road to habitual drug-taking may start with the desire for 'arousal jag' which stimulants like amphetamines can offer. For the very anxious it may begin with the discovery that barbiturates or alcohol enable them to cope with social situations that would otherwise be agony to bear. Those who go on to swell the ranks of the 'hard' drug addicts may have severe personality problems traceable to a variety of events in their life histories.

Because the factors that may lead to drug dependency are so diverse, it is not to be expected that any particular kind of individual can be identified as the 'addict type'. This has not deterred research workers in this area from trying to isolate the personality characteristics which may predispose certain people to become dependent on drugs. Attention has naturally been focussed on those who are severely addicted and here, as anticipated, we find a high proportion of deviant personality types. Both chronic alcoholics and confirmed narcotic addicts are commonly described as immature, excessively dependent individuals, often sexually inadequate and highly disturbed in their relationships with others. Unfortunately, this is true of many psychiatrically ill people and any sample of drug addicts will probably be found to contain almost the full range of mental disorder. The only feature common to all addicts is that drugs enable them to deal with one or other of many deficiencies in their own personalities. By escaping into a drug-induced world of make-believe they can avoid facing the harsh reality of personal inadequacy. One theory to explain why the addict seeks this particular way out of his psychological problems is that drugs enable him to make at least a reasonable adjustment to life, where none at all would otherwise be possible. According to this view, drugs actually serve a useful purpose by preventing the disturbed personality breaking down into more severe psychotic illness. Peter Laurie discusses such a view in his recent Penguin on drug addiction [42]. In doing so, he draws particularly on the opinions of Ronald Laing and the notion that some addicts seem to be similar in personality to the young schizophrenic. According to Laing, and others who regard schizophrenia as psychological in origin, both types of person are said to have similar family backgrounds. Both, it is suggested, commonly come from homes in which they had strong but ambivalent relationships with their mothers, but where the fathers were ineffectual. Laurie concludes that, as an alternative to the schizophrenic reaction which this kind of environment is said to produce, some individuals may resort to drugs. The hypothesis is an interesting one though concrete evidence to support it is lacking at the present time. Even the psychogenic theory of schizophrenia itself is unproven and the family factors emphasized by Laing may not be specific to schizophrenia at all but, for all we know, may occur in other abnormal personalities. Of course, it could still be true that, as Laurie suggests, drugs help some individuals keep at bay a developing psychotic illness, however caused. It is probable, however, that this is only one of many different kinds of unpleasant reality from which those addicted to drugs are trying to escape. For the very diversity of subjective effects that drugs can produce, from sedative to stimulant to hallucinogenic, almost matches the variety of personalities who can become dependent on them. A still unsolved problem in psychiatry is why some people use drugs and others find alternative ways of dealing with the tensions within themselves.

Few readers, unless they work in a psychiatric clinic, will have come face to face with a heroin or amphetamine addict. Some may not even have met an alcoholic. For most members of society severe drug addiction is something that lies below the surface, heatedly discussed in the press and on television but actually indulged in by other people. This complacent notion of 'we' and 'they' is misguided. For, as I have already emphasized, medically recognized addiction is only the pathological end-point of a continuum of drug-taking that involves us all. Even the most upright of citizens have their chemical comforters, most of which are psychologically harmless when taken in small quantities. Indeed, they usually provide a pleasant relaxation from the daily grind. Dependence on them is rarely a problem either. It is betrayed only by a flicker of irritability if the coffee is late, the pub closed, or the cigarette packet empty. Nevertheless, even this moderate use of drugs has posed problems of its own for society. Unlike drug addiction, these problems are encountered daily by everyone and from time to time have prompted society to introduce restrictions or propaganda in an attempt to control excessive drug consumption by the ordinary individual. In the case of cigarettes, of course, the dangers have been identified as those of physical disease not always connected with the nicotine that partly drives the smoking habit. As far as behaviour is concerned, it is again alcohol that exposes society at large to its greatest hazard; not because we are all likely to become alcoholic – only some of us will – but because of the reduced psychological efficiency that even a single dose of alcohol can produce. The consequence, that of increased accident risk, would be less serious if only a few people were involved or the drinker alone were affected. Unfortunately, this is not the case, for one person under the influence of alcohol may endanger others who are perfectly sober.

The question of drugs in relation to public safety has been discussed mainly with respect to alcohol and car-driving and I will return to that in a moment. It is sometimes forgotten, however, that there are some equally important, though less obvious, aspects to the problem. Not all accidents occur on the roads. Some happen in the home. Others, sometimes quite dangerous ones, occur in industry and it has been variously estimated that between ten and twenty per cent of accidents there involve workers who have been drinking. Even if the lower figure were more nearly correct it would still represent a substantial loss of man-hours directly attributable to alcohol. And, of course, many people carry out their daily activities under the influence of drugs other than alcohol. In a recent survey by the Automobile Association in Great Britain it was found that one out of every seven drivers interviewed had taken a drug of one kind or another during the previous twenty-four hours [69]. The AA comments that, if its sample is representative, then two million people in Britain drive daily under the influence of drugs that can potentially impair driving skill. What is worse, most of the drivers interviewed were unaware of the risks involved, few of those taking prescribed medicines having been told by their doctors that it may be unsafe to drive. However, on the roads it is not always the drinking (or drugged) driver who is at fault. The inebriated pedestrian can sometimes place the driver in a dangerous situation where it is impossible to avoid an accident. It is interesting, for example, that in a survey of fatalities occurring over a recent Christmas and New Year period, the Road Research Laboratory found that 30 per cent of pedestrians killed on the roads in England and Wales had evidence of alcohol in their blood. In Scotland the figure was a staggering 64 per cent, the proportion of pedestrians who died there with alcohol in their blood actually being *greater* than that for drivers who were killed [5].

Because of the size of the problem it is understandable that most attention, however, has been paid to alcohol and driving, that highly complex skill which all but the most grossly disabled are free to pursue after an eyesight test and a supervised run round a familiar and well-practised route. Unfortunately, even the most proficient and alert can sometimes make mistakes. If they have been drinking, the risk of an accident is inevitably further increased, for like most other skills driving can be disrupted by alcohol. The evidence to support this conclusion scarcely needs to be enumerated in detail here. It comes from many sources. Even at the end of the last century experimental psychologists had shown that alcohol impairs simple responses like reaction time. Since then the effect of alcohol on almost every other piece of human behaviour has been investigated. Although the results are not always consistent from one study to the next, in general alcohol lives up to its classification as a depressant drug. In order to discover how alcohol affects driving itself some research has looked at the behaviour of people either actually controlling a car or performing on car-simulators. The latter are specially designed mock cars something like, though more elaborate than, the ones used by some driving schools to introduce their pupils to the basic principles of vehicle-handling before sending them out on the roads. Used in the experimental laboratory, they have the advantage that different components of driving skill can each be studied separately and measured accurately. An important experiment using such a device was carried out some years ago by Professor Drew and his colleagues in collaboration with the Road Research Laboratory [18]. They gave volunteer subjects several sessions of 'driving' on a car-simulator after either a placebo drink or after one of a series of graded doses of alcohol, the largest being roughly equivalent to three pints of beer or three double whiskies. Their results showed quite clearly that accuracy, speed, and handling of driving controls were all significantly impaired by alcohol, the amount of error becoming more pronounced as the dose-level increased.

Another kind of evidence for the disruptive effects of alcohol on driving comes from the statistics on road accidents. These are of two kinds. One concerns the frequency with which confirmed alcoholics have accidents. Not surprisingly, it has been found that such people are much more at risk, and place others more at risk, than the ordinary individual. One American study, carried out in the San Francisco Bay area of California, showed that alcoholics were four-and-a-half times more likely to die in a road accident [8]. They were, incidentally, also more likely to die following some other incident – even smoking in bed. The notion that the heavy drinker is somehow immune because he has acquired a tremendous tolerance for alcohol is therefore a dangerous misconception. While it may be true that in the experimental laboratory the alcoholic is less impaired, dose for dose, than normal, in real life his drinking habits are unfortunately not so regulated. For, as Professor E. J. Wayne astutely pointed out at a recent symposium on road safey, 'after all, people do not drink to obtain a given blood level of alcohol but to achieve euphoria' [71].

Of course, by no means all accidents involving alcohol are caused by chronic alcoholics and the main facts implicating the drug as a disruptive influence on driving have come from the general road accident statistics. Some of the evidence is indirect, such as the finding that the frequency of accidents increases sharply at certain times of day, particularly after the pubs have closed, or at certain times of year, such as Christmas, when drinking is excessive. Other, more direct, evidence has been obtained from special studies of the drinking habits or blood alcohol levels of people involved in road accidents. The most comprehensive study of this kind was carried out several years ago in the United States by a team of workers led by Professor Borkenstein of Indiana University [6]. They set out to investigate the accidents occurring over a one-year period in the city of Grand Rapids, Michigan. During the year of the survey, 9,359 drivers were involved in accidents. Of these nearly 6,000 were interviewed and asked to provide personal information which included age, marital and occupational status, drinking habits, and annual driving mileage. In addition, a breath sample was taken from each driver and later analysed to give an estimate of his blood alcohol level at the time. This accident-involved group was compared with a second, control, group of drivers who had not had accidents but whose exposure to that risk was similar. Control drivers were obtained by randomly stopping passing motorists at predetermined times and places and asking them to

provide a breath sample and the same information as that
gathered from accident drivers. It was then possible to determine
how the relative accident rate of the two groups varied according
to the different items of information collected. This was done by
working out an 'accident-involvement index' based on the
relative frequency with which accident and control drivers showed
a particular characteristic. In the case of the breath analysis data,
changes in accident involvement index could then be related to
variations in blood alcohol level. These results are illustrated in
Figure 9.1, which shows the accident-involvement index plotted
against increasing blood alcohol level. A word about the two axes
in the figure will help the reader to interpret it. In the case of the
accident-involvement index, a positive value indicates that the

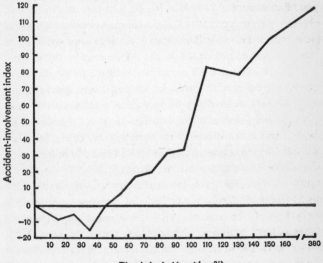

Fig. 9.1. Results of the Grand Rapids study, showing how the risk of
having a road accident (accident involvement index) changes as the blood
alcohol concentration increases. The small *drop* in accident risk at very
low blood alcohol levels is discussed further in the text.

(From results reported by R. F. Borkenstein. Reported here with his
permission.)

risk of having an accident is that much greater with, than without, a given level of alcohol in the blood. Negative values suggest the converse, while a zero index shows that the accident risk is unaltered at that particular blood alcohol level. The latter itself is recorded as milligrammes of alcohol per 100 millilitres of blood, which is usually abbreviated to mg/100 ml or mg per cent. This particular index is one of several ways in which the concentration of alcohol in the blood can be expressed, but it is the one most commonly used for medico-legal purposes.

Returning to Figure 9.1, it can be seen that with rising blood alcohol there is a rapidly increasing risk of being involved in a road accident. The danger becomes particularly great above 100 mg per cent, a blood alcohol figure which would be reached by a man of average height drinking five pints of beer, or five double whiskies, an hour or so after a normal meal. As one would expect, the details of Professor Borkenstein's findings were rather more complicated than is shown in Figure 9.1. One odd result is illustrated in the diagram itself, namely the tendency for accident risk actually to *decrease* at low blood alcohol levels. Furthermore, other driver characteristics besides alcohol consumption were also associated with accident involvement. I will come back to some of these points later. In the meantime, we can quite safely conclude that the evidence against alcohol as an important contributor to road accidents is unassailable.

It is on the basis of this fact that many countries have introduced legislation setting upper limits of blood or urine alcohol beyond which the motorist can be prosecuted. In the United States and in Scandinavia such laws have been in operation for a number of years. In October 1967 Great Britain finally followed suit through the efforts of our erstwhile lady Minister of Transport, Mrs Barbara Castle, who, without disrespect, may be said to have pulled it off by dint of 'breath, blood, and urine'. As no British road user should need reminding, the upper blood alcohol level she and her advisers fixed was 80 mg. per cent. This figure is higher than that adopted by some countries, Norway for example penalizing drivers found to have blood alcohol levels above 50 mg. per cent. It is, on the other hand, lower than that used in some American states. The limit of 80 mg. per cent was chosen in Britain because it was felt to be low enough to make a significant contribution to road safety, yet high enough to avoid injustice being done to individual motorists; for it was considered that at that level almost everybody's driving skill would be noticeably impaired.

On its introduction the 'Breathalyzer' gave rise to fierce controversy about its fairness and to many apocryphal stories about how it could be dodged. (One such story, which I think I can repeat without endangering the road safety campaign, concerns a man who always carries a bottle of urine around with him – suitably warmed and alcohol-free, of course.) More seriously, one of the main arguments advanced against the 'Breathalyzer' is that it fails to take account of the variable effects on behaviour that drugs can produce. How relevant is this objection? It is certainly true, as we saw in an earlier chapter, that many factors, physical, psychological, and social, can modify the action of drugs, so that their precise effects may be difficult to predict from one situation or one individual to the next. This variability applies as much to the drinking driver as to any other person taking drugs. When looked at from the point of view of road accidents the problem becomes an extremely complex one, as some of Professor Borkenstein's other findings illustrate. The results of the Grand Rapids study were later re-analysed by the Road Research Laboratory which examined the interaction between blood alcohol level and other driver characteristics tabulated by Professor Borkenstein [1]. It was found that the relative contribution of alcohol to accident-involvement depended on the presence or absence of other features in the driver. Thus, the risk of an accident was generally lower in middle-aged men of high occupational and educational status who drank fairly frequently and drove a high annual mileage. It is this group that appears to account for the surprising finding, commented upon earlier, that at low blood alcohol levels – up to about 40 mg. per cent – accident risk actually falls. How we explain the result is a different matter. The most probable reason is that in the experienced driver who, say, calls in for a quick drink, perhaps on his way home from work, a small dose of alcohol acts as a mild tranquillizer and has the beneficial effect of relieving the tensions and anxieties of the day. Added to this is the fact that such people may afterwards take extra care because they will be more than usually aware of the dangers of alcohol. Of course, it should be remembered that the reduced accident risk found in the Grand Rapids study occurred only at *low* blood alcohol levels, well below the British statutory figure of 80 mg. per cent. Both Professor Borkenstein and the Road Research Laboratory emphasize strongly that, as blood alcohol level rises, so the contribution of other driver characteristics to accident risk assumes less and less importance. Furthermore, even at very low alcohol levels certain individuals are more than usually prone to have an accident. For example, despite the average trend, teenage drivers studied by Professor Borkenstein had an enormously increased accident involvement index when their blood alcohol levels fell within the range 10–49 mg. per cent.

An extension of the argument about the variable effects of alcohol is that there are wide differences in tolerance of the drug, either natural or acquired. Again it is true, as we have already seen, that some people are less affected by sedative drugs than others, the variation in susceptibility being partly a biologically determined characteristic. Most of the experimental work on this problem has involved the use of barbiturate drugs, but at least one study has looked at alcohol itself. And indeed sedation thresholds obtained using ethyl alcohol vary as much as those found with barbiturates. Furthermore, the correlations with personality are very similar, anxious individuals being most tolerant of alcohol. Does this mean that some highly resistant people are being unfairly penalized by the new legislation? In theory it probably does, though, as I have already mentioned, the blood alcohol level of 80 mg. per cent was deliberately chosen in order to avoid putting more than a very small proportion of the population in that category. The real question is whether the figure decided upon is too *high*. Human nature being what it is the loudest protests about the 'Breathalyzer' have come from those who think, rightly or wrongly, that they can hold their booze better than most. People with a poor stomach for alcohol are much less ready to advertise the fact. These, as we know from previous chapters, tend to be rather extraverted, psychopathic or hysterical individuals. Regrettably they often also tend to be the people who drink deepest and drive hardest. Extraverted drivers are therefore likely to be doubly at risk. Take just one example, that of motorway driving. Here the driver is subjected to long, boring stretches at the wheel, with little to relieve the monotony. We know from experimental studies that under these conditions a person's vigilance is likely to falter. This is much more likely to happen under sedative drugs and in extraverted people. The two together could be a fatal combination.

Fortunately, the hard-drinking extravert may be protected to some extent by an increased tolerance of alcohol acquired through frequent indulgence in the drug. A less obvious form of protection may be provided by the extravert's body weight or body build. It is known that there are small but consistent relationships between personality and these physical characteristics. The stockiness of the extravert may contribute to a lower absorption rate of alcohol and in a small way cancel out his basically poorer resistance to the drug. Of course, neither safeguard, acquired tolerance nor increased body weight, will be so obvious in the young person and it is almost certain that the point at which some individuals in this high-risk group become severely impaired by alcohol is well below the statutory limit of 80 mg. per cent.

The crux of all of these arguments about the 'Breathalyzer' is that the tests the police are empowered to use only tell them how much alcohol the body tissues contain. They do not tell them the degree to which the individual's behaviour is actually disrupted.

Naturally, there is little doubt that a driver is totally incapable if he is found weaving from one side of the road to the other. Technically, however, if they suspect that a motorist has been drinking the police can stop him for a purely minor offence, such as a broken stoplight. While such a system may be reasonably fair in practice, it does not help to counter the objection that blood alcohol only provides an indirect measure of a person's inability to drive. Unfortunately, the alternative would be impossibly complex and the subject of even greater controversy. That would be to equip the police with suitable apparatus that would allow them to measure a driver's skill as well as his blood alcohol level. Such apparatus would either be so simple it would be useless or so elaborate as to be impracticable. It would, for example, be perfectly feasible to measure reaction time with a high degree of accuracy; but reaction time as such bears very little relationship to driving skill. The use of more complicated equipment, such as car-simulators permanently installed in police stations, would be nearer to the applied psychologist's dream of justice. The mind boggles at the technical, administrative, and legal problems that they would introduce.

For the time being, at any rate, the measurement of tissue alcohol levels would therefore appear to provide the most accurate and convenient method of detecting the drunken driver. The problem of variability we shall have to accept and live with or, if it proves necessary, deal with by amendments within the existing format of legislation. Even here some of the alternatives would either be unacceptable or unworkable. To ban road users from drinking altogether would go so much against cultural tradition and cause so much public outcry that no government would dare to try it. On the other hand, a sliding scale of guilt, a sort of motorist's means test based on the sedation threshold, would be as laughable as individual speed limits tailored to suit the skills of different drivers. The third alternative, lowering the statutory level of blood alcohol, might be a real possibility. This would probably cause even greater protest than the present

'Breathalyzer' law but, if it were introduced, the price to be paid by those highly tolerant of alcohol would be small when set against the saving of human life. For after all, we are exhorted not to drink and drive at all.

Whether it becomes necessary to revise the present blood alcohol limit for drivers will be decided to some extent by the long-term accident statistics of the future. The new legislation has been operative in Britain for such a short time that any conclusions at the moment about its effectiveness would be premature. However, its immediate impact on the accident rate has been evaluated by the Ministry of Transport [52]. Figure 9.2 shows the incidence of deaths and serious injuries on British roads during the six months after the introduction of the 'Breathalyzer', compared with the equivalent six-month period a year earlier. It can be seen that for the period under review the 'Breathalyzer' produced a general fall in the number of serious accidents. More significant, perhaps, is the fact that a good deal of the improvement occurred at peak accident times when drivers are likely to have been drinking, namely on Friday and Saturday evenings. Over the whole period there was a twenty per cent fall in the number of deaths in road accidents, which in absolute figures represents a drop from 4,295 to 3,440 people, a saving of 855 lives. This improvement in the road casualty figures is encouraging, though it is certainly an overestimate of the saving we might expect in the future, since the public inevitably took special care to avoid drinking and driving immediately after the new law came into force. In fact, more recent monthly accident statistics suggest that motorists are now beginning to relax their efforts and the casualty rate has risen again.

However satisfying this small improvement in the accident figures may be it is still a sad fact that far too many people are killed or injured on the roads each year – over 3,000 deaths in six months even with a restriction on alcohol consumption. It is probable that some further saving could have been achieved had the Government fixed the statutory blood alcohol limit lower than

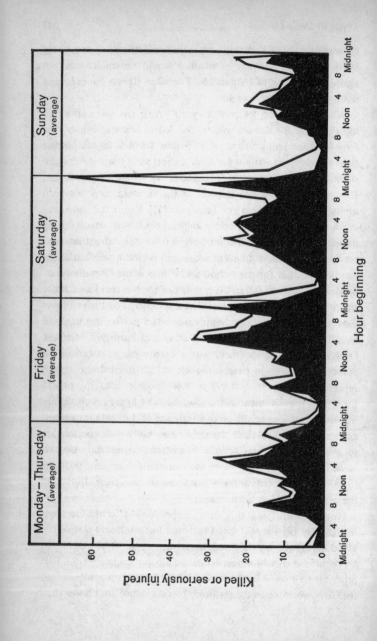

80 mg. per cent. However, legislation of this kind inevitably follows a law of diminishing returns and the bulk of the accident statistics would remain untouched. The reason is painfully obvious; namely that the most important contributory factors in road accidents are those most difficult to control. They are human ones, originating within the driver himself. To try and analyse this difficult subject in detail would take us far beyond the scope of the book; but a word or two about it in relation to drugs may help the reader to view the problem of drink and driving against the wider background of driver behaviour in general.

All of us know the emotional attitudes that can lead to road accidents: the feeling of aggression when thwarted by another driver or of impatience in a traffic snarl-up. Most people manage to control their feelings most of the time or, if they do lapse, survive through a combination of luck and reserve skill. In some individuals, however, several antisocial attitudes may occur together and the feelings associated with them be triggered off more quickly than normal. Such people, especially if they are young and inexperienced, are often found to be accident 're-peaters' and probably make up the majority of accident-prone drivers. Even when sober they frequently place others, and themselves, in danger. When drunk the risks may be enormously increased. We have already seen how at a simple biological level – the extravert's poor tolerance of monotony – the depressant action of alcohol may interact with existing personality characteristics.

Here, however, we are dealing with the much more complex

Fig. 9.2. Average number of deaths and serious injuries on the road at different times of day and week before and after introduction of the 'Breathalyzer'. A comparison is made between the period October 1966–March 1967 (white area) and October 1967–March 1968 (black area). Note particularly the reduction in serious accidents during the 'drinking hours', late Friday and Saturday evenings.

(Adapted from a diagram published by the Ministry of Transport.)

problem of the driver's psychopathology and how on occasions alcohol may bring out the worst in people. The problem is thrown into relief by a recent American study of psychological attitudes associated with road accidents in a group of emotionally disturbed psychiatric patients [54]. The sample was divided into two groups; those who were alcoholic and those who were not. For all patients a record was made of the number of road accidents they had been involved in over a fixed period, the incidents being listed according to whether the individual had previously been drinking or not. Each patient was also subjected to an extensive psychiatric interview in order to elicit emotional attitudes which it was felt might predict accident potential. As far as the frequency of accidents was concerned, it was found that alcoholics when drunk had many more than non-alcoholics; but when sober both groups were equally accident-prone. More interesting, however, were the relationships between personality and accident potential. It was shown that the tendency to have a traffic accident was highly correlated with certain emotional attitudes, particularly persecutory and aggressive feelings and depressive ideas, such as despondency and suicidal preoccupation. A combination of such traits was able to predict accident potential with a high degree of accuracy, much more so than the single fact that the individual might previously have been drinking. These relationships with personality were true of both alcoholics and non-alcoholics, though in the former they were more marked. The authors of the study concluded that in the alcoholic driver we see an extreme example of the interplay between intoxication and certain deleterious personality traits. Thus, alcohol will have two effects. It will release emotional attitudes which, even when the individual is sober, may predispose him to have an accident. At the same time it will disrupt his driving skill, making it even more difficult for him to take avoiding action in the face of emergency.

The reader may perhaps object that the study of psychiatric misfits I have just described is scarcely typical of the average person's experience of alcohol. That is true. A similar objection could be raised against many of the examples of drug effects quoted in this book, some of which have involved mentally disturbed people, others normal volunteer subjects taking part in laboratory experiments far removed from real life. Yet no one who has reflected on the results of these studies can fail to have seen something of their own psychology in the variety of mental states that drugs can produce. The drugs we have been concerned with here sometimes exaggerate or distort; sometimes they merely excite or calm. But always they act through psychological mechanisms that exist in all of us to a greater or lesser degree.

In Conclusion 10

It has been said that advances in knowledge often occur at the edges of scientific disciplines where two or more specialties overlap and when individuals from adjacent fields of research join forces to study a common problem. As this book has shown, psychopharmacology is a good example of such collaborative endeavour, for it is a body of knowledge shared by a mongrel breed of scientists whose original training may have been in any one of a number of fields, including psychology, neurophysiology, psychiatry, or, of course, pharmacology. In the foregoing chapters we have seen how, as psychopharmacologists, they go about studying the way drugs affect behaviour or using drugs as special techniques for understanding behaviour. I have tried throughout to draw attention to areas of ignorance as well as areas of knowledge. For, although there have been great advances in psychopharmacology over the past twenty years – indeed without them it could not have emerged as an independent discipline – there are many facts about behaviour and many drugs still to be discovered. Thus, although we can render normal people temporarily insane with drugs, we have little idea as yet how to make the naturally psychotic well again. Nor do we know why some mentally disturbed individuals crave the oblivion (or excitement) of drugs, while others, equally sick, are indifferent to them. In another sphere, the psychopharmacologist can accurately describe and measure the behavioural and overt physiological changes that occur when someone is sedated. But what is happening in the brain at the same time is still largely a matter of surmise.

These, and numerous other, questions which will have occurred to the reader throughout the book, provide the future challenge for psychopharmacologists. In answering them psychopharmacology and its sister sciences will further extend man's understanding of himself and his ability to control and direct behaviour by chemical means. In the future, as now, much of the effort will be directed towards finding ways of relieving mental suffering, for this has traditionally been the springboard for research in psychopharmacology. In the process, however, many fundamental facts about human behaviour in general will be unearthed and the practical usefulness of psychotropic drugs will certainly extend beyond the psychiatric clinic. If one such application had to be chosen from the many possibilities it would be from the field of learning and memory, a new but rapidly growing aspect of psychopharmacology. The plasticity of human behaviour is one of its most vital characteristics and the eventual discovery of new drugs that will affect quite specific features of the learning process has exciting implications for the future. For example, as envisaged in an earlier chapter, psychotropic drugs might well find a place in education as an aid to learning and, more distantly, in the arrest of the memory loss characteristic of old age.

The benefits that future developments in psychopharmacology bring will not be won without the creation of new problems for society or the exacerbation of existing ones. Possibly the most ironic is that of drug addiction, which has already caused psychopharmacology to expand its own boundaries in order to search for effective cures, some of which involve the use of drugs. Perhaps future research will find a more radical solution by synthesizing a new class of drugs that are physically harmless but which still satisfy man's age-old desire for chemicals that transport him to other planes of experience. Or maybe greater knowledge of man himself will enable him to find other sources of satisfaction, if only in the form of a universally effective placebo.

In the meantime all sectors of society are going through a crisis of uncertainty about drugs. Doctors who prescribe them professionally are becoming increasingly troubled by the variety of remedies offered by the pharmaceutical companies; though factual evidence about the effectiveness of many new drugs is often deplorably meagre. Many patients who take drugs prescribed for them are more than dimly aware that their problems are too complicated to be solved by a pretty-looking capsule. Yet they continue to take them because they find that, temporarily, they work – or at least they believe they do. The confusion about drugs is crystallized most clearly, however, in society's attitudes towards illicit drug-taking. At one extreme, permissive elements in society demand greater freedom to use (or abuse) their bodies as they wish. At the other extreme, punitive attitudes motivate the cry for greater legal sanctions on some forms of drug-taking. Both viewpoints are equally irrational. Many drugs are highly dangerous and rigid controls over them can only be for the good of the community. But whether action of this kind is demanded or not may often depend as much on a drug's respectability as upon the risks inherent in its use. Is it not illogical that, technically, house-owners can be prosecuted because someone else, unbeknown to them, smokes marihuana on their premises; while any one among us can quite legally drink himself under the table in the company of the local magistrate?

At present psychopharmacology is only just beginning to offer society a more rational basis for the way it deals with drugs, whether taken legally or illegally. But one thing is certain.

Further progress will depend as much upon increasing our knowledge of drugs as upon deepening our understanding of people. For that, after all, is what psychopharmacology is all about.

Further Reading

For specialist articles on particular topics in psychopharmacology the reader is directed to the psychological and psychiatric journals, all of which regularly cover various aspects of drug effects. In addition the journal *Psychopharmacologia* is entirely devoted to experimental studies of drugs; while the *Quarterly Journal of Studies on Alcohol* publishes articles on alcohol from both the experimental and addictive points of view. Recent advances in psychopharmacology are regularly brought together at the international congresses of the Collegium Internationale Neuropsychopharmacologicum, the proceedings of which are published in book form every few years.

For the experimentally minded the following general publications are suggested:

TROUTON, D. and EYSENCK, H. J. 'The effects of drugs on behaviour'. In EYSENCK, H. J. (Ed.), *Handbook of Abnormal Psychology*, Pitman, 1960.

UHR, L. and MILLER, J. G. (Eds.), *Drugs and Behaviour*, Wiley, New York, 1960.

For the more general reader the following book gives a good overview of current trends in psychopharmacology:

JOYCE, C. R. B. (Ed.), *Psychopharmacology, Dimensions and Perspectives*, Tavistock Publications, 1968.

Finally, the following publications are suggested for those wishing to read more about some of the special topics discussed in the book:

(Chapter 2) BEECHER, H. K. *Measurement of Subjective Responses*, Oxford University Press, 1959.
(Chapter 5) COHEN, S. *Drugs of Hallucination*, Secker & Warburg, 1965.
(Chapter 7) CLARIDGE, G. S. *Personality and Arousal*, Pergamon, 1967.
(Chapter 9) LAURIE, Peter. *Drugs. Medical, Psychological and Social Facts*, Penguin Books, 1967.

References

1. 'Alcohol and road accidents'. Ministry of Transport, Road Research Laboratory Report No. 6, 1966.
2. BAKER, A. A. and THORPE, J. G., 'Placebo response'. *Archives of Neurology and Psychiatry*, vol. 78, 1957, pp. 57–60.
3. BEECH, H. R., *Changing Man's Behaviour*. Penguin Books, 1969.
4. BERLIN, L., GUTHRIE, T., WEIDER, A., GOODELL, H. and WOLFF, H. G., 'Studies in human cerebral function: the effects of mescaline and lysergic acid on cerebral processes pertinent to creative activity'. *Journal of Nervous and Mental Disease*, vol. 122, 1955, pp. 487–91.
5. 'Blood alcohol levels in road accident fatalities occurring in Gt Britain during December, 1964 and January, 1965'. Ministry of Transport, Road Research Laboratory Report No. 32, 1966.
6. BORKENSTEIN, R. F., CROWTHER, R. F., SCHUMATE, R. P., ZIEL, W. B., and ZYLMAN, R., 'The role of the drinking driver in traffic accidents'. Indiana University, Department of Police Administration, 1964.

7. BRADLEY, P. B., 'The central action of certain drugs in relation to the reticular formation of the brain'. In: JASPER, H. H., *et al.* (Eds.), *Reticular Formation of the Brain*, Churchill, 1957.

8. BRENNER, B., 'Alcoholism and fatal accidents'. *Quarterly Journal of Studies on Alcohol*, vol. 28, 1967, pp. 517–28.

9. BURCH, N. R. and GREINER, T. H., 'A bioelectric scale of human alertness: concurrent recordings of the EEG and GSR'. *Psychiatric Research Reports of the American Psychiatric Association*, no. 12, 1960, pp. 183–93.

10. CALLAWAY, E. and DEMBO, D., 'Narrowed attention'. *Archives of Neurology and Psychiatry*, vol. 79, 1958, pp. 74–90.

11. CHAPMAN, J., 'The early symptoms of schizophrenia'. *British Journal of Psychiatry*, vol. 112, 1966, pp. 225–51.

12. CLARIDGE, G. S., 'The effects of meprobamate on the performance of a five-choice reaction time task'. *Journal of Mental Science*, vol. 107, 1961, pp. 590–602.

13. CLARIDGE, G. S. and HERRINGTON, R. N., 'Sedation threshold, personality and the theory of neurosis'. *Journal of Mental Science*, vol. 106, 1960, pp. 1568–83.

14. CLARIDGE, G. S. and HUME, W I., 'Comparison of effects of dexamphetamine and LSD-25 on perceptual and autonomic function'. *Perceptual and Motor Skills*, vol. 23, 1966, pp. 456–8.

15. CORSSEN, G. and DOMINO, E. F., 'Visually evoked responses in man: a method for measuring cerebral effects of preanaesthetic medication'. *Anesthesiology*, vol. 25, 1964, pp. 330–41.

16. CROMIE, B. W. and INGRAM, I. M., 'A pilot study on a limitation of identical placebos in cross-over trials'. *Journal of Therapeutics and Clinical Research*, vol. 1, 1967, pp. 9–11.

17. DAVIES, M. H., CLARIDGE, G. S. and WAWMAN, R. J., 'Sedation threshold, autonomic lability and the excitation-inhibition theory of personality. III. The blood pressure response to an adrenaline antagonist as a measure of autonomic lability'. *British Journal of Psychiatry*, vol. 109, 1963, pp. 558–67.

18. DREW, G. C., COLQUHOUN, W. P., and LONG, H. A., 'Effect of small doses of alcohol on a skill resembling driving'. *MRC Memorandum No. 38*, H.M.S.O., 1959.

19. 'Drug addiction'. Number 25 in a series of papers on current health problems, Office of Health Economics, 1967.

20. EVANS, W. O. and DAVIS, K. E., 'Dose-response effects of secobarbital on human memory'. *Psychopharmacologia*, vol. 14, 1969, pp. 46–61.

21. EYSENCK, H. J., CASEY, S., and TROUTON, D. S., 'Drugs and personality. II. The effect of stimulant and depressant drugs on continuous work'. *Journal of Mental Science*, vol. 103, 1957, pp. 645–9.

22. 'Fellini's daily miracle'. Federico Fellini talks with Michael Caen. *Envoy*, vol. 1, 1968, mid-March/mid-April, pp. 14–21.

23. FÉRÉ, C., *The Pathology of Emotions*. English edition, translated by R. Park, The University Press, London, 1899.

24. FISHER. S. and FISHER, R. L., 'Placebo response and acquiescence'. *Psychopharmacologia*, vol. 4, 1963, pp. 298-301.

25. FRANKENHAEUSER, M., JAERPE, G., SVAN, H., and WRANGS-JOE, B., 'Psychophysiological reactions to two different placebo treatments'. *Scandinavian Journal of Psychology*, vol. 4, 1963, pp. 245–50.

26. FRANKENHAEUSER, M., POST, B., HAGDAHL, R., and WRANGS-JOE, B., 'Effects of a depressant drug as modified by experimentally-induced expectation'. *Perceptual and Motor Skills*, vol. 18, 1964, pp. 513–22.

27. FRANKS, C. M. and TROUTON, D., 'Effects of amobarbital sodium and dexamphetamine sulphate in the conditioning of the eyeblink response'. *Journal of Comparative and Physiological Psychology*, vol. 51, 1958, pp. 220–22.

28. GLASS, H. B., 'Genetic aspects of adaptability'. In: *Genetics and the Inheritance of Integrated Neurological and Psychiatric Patterns*. Proceedings for Research in Nervous and Mental Disease, vol. 33, Williams and Wilkins, Baltimore, 1954.

29. HERRINGTON, R. N., 'The effect of amphetamine on a serial reaction task'. *Psychopharmacologia*, vol. 12, 1967, pp. 50–57.

30. HERRINGTON, R. N. and CLARIDGE, G. S., 'Sedation threshold and Archimedes' spiral after-effect in early psychosis'. *Journal of Psychiatric Research*, vol. 3, 1965, pp. 159–70.

31. HILL, H. E., BELLEVILLE, R. E., and WIKLER, A., 'Motivational determinants in modification of behaviour by morphine and pentobarbital'. *Archives of Neurology and Psychiatry*, vol. 77, 1957, pp. 28–35.

32. HOUSE, Jackson, 'How hallucinations built a hospital'. *Canadian Weekly*, 9–15 January 1965.

33. JARVIK, M., 'The influence of drugs on memory'. In Ciba Symposium, *Animal Behaviour and Drug Action*, Churchill, 1964.

34. KALIN, R., 'Effects of alcohol on memory'. *Journal of Abnormal and Social Psychology*, vol. 69, 1964, pp. 635–41.

35. KEY, B. J., 'Effect of LSD-25 on potentials evoked in specific sensory pathways'. *British Medical Bulletin*, vol. 21, 1965, pp. 30–35.

36. KEY, B. J., 'The effect of drugs on discrimination and sensory generalization of auditory stimuli in cats'. *Psychopharmacologia*, vol. 2, 1961, pp. 352–63.

37. KEY, B. J., 'The effect of LSD-25 on the interaction between conditioned and non-conditioned stimuli in a simple avoidance situation'. *Psychopharmacologia*, vol. 6, 1964, pp. 319–26.

38. KLERMAN, G. L., DiMASCIO, A., GREENBLATT, M., and RINKEL, M., 'The influence of specific personality patterns on the reactions to psychotropic agents'. In MASSERMAN, J. H. (Ed.), *Biological Psychiatry*, Grune and Stratton, New York, 1959.

39. KNOWLES, J. B. and LUCAS, C. J., 'Experimental studies of the placebo response'. *Journal of Mental Science*, vol. 106, 1960, pp. 231–40.

40. KRISHNAMOORTI, S. R. and SHAGASS, C., 'Some psychological test correlates of sedation threshold'. In WORTIS, J. (Ed.), *Recent Advances in Biological Psychiatry*, vol. 6, Plenum Press, New York, 1964.

41. LADER, M. H. and WING, L., *Physiological Measures, Sedative Drugs, and Morbid Anxiety*. Oxford University Press, 1966.

42. LAURIE, Peter, *Drugs*, Penguin Books, 1967.

43. LEHMANN, H. E. and KNIGHT, M. A., 'Placebo-proneness and placebo resistance of different psychological functions'. *Psychiatric Quarterly*, vol. 34, 1960, pp. 505–16.

44. LIEBERT, R. S., WERNER, H. and WAPNER, S., 'Studies in the effect of lysergic acid diethylamide (LSD-25)'. *Archives of Neurology and Psychiatry*, vol. 79, 1958, pp. 580–84.

45. LINTON, H. B. and LANGS, R. J., 'Subjective reactions to lysergic acid diethylamide (LSD-25)', *Archives of General Psychiatry*, vol. 6, 1962, pp. 352–68.

46. MCPEAKE, J. D., and DiMASCIO, A., 'Drug–personality

interaction in the learning of a nonsense syllable task'. *Journal of Psychiatric Research*, vol. 3, 1965, pp. 105–11.

47. MIRSKY, A. F. and ROSVOLD, H. E., 'The use of psychoactive drugs as a neuropsychological tool in studies of attention in man'. In UHR, L. and MILLER, J. G. (Eds.), *Drugs and Behaviour*, Wiley, New York, 1960.

48. OSWALD, I., 'Some psychophysiological features of human sleep'. *Progress in Brain Research*, vol. 18, Elsevier, Amsterdam, 1965.

49. PARK, L. C. and COUI, L., 'Nonblind placebo trial'. *Archives of General Psychiatry*, vol. 12, 1965, pp. 336–45.

50. PEREZ-REYES, M. and COCHRANE, C., 'Differences in sodium thiopental susceptibility of depressed patients as evidenced by the galvanic skin reflex inhibition threshold'. *Journal of Psychiatric Research*, vol. 5, 1967, pp. 335–47.

51. REED, C. F. and WITT, P. N., 'Factors contributing to unexpected reactions in two human drug–placebo experiments'. *Confinia Psychiatrica*, vol. 8, 1965, pp. 57–68.

52. 'Road Accidents 1967'. Ministry of Transport, H.M.S.O., 1968.

53. RODNIGHT, E. and GOOCH, R. N., 'A new method for the determination of individual differences in susceptibility to a depressant drug'. In EYSENCK, H. J. (Ed.), *Experiments with Drugs*, Pergamon, 1963.

54. SELZER, M. L., PAYNE, C. E., WESTERVELT, F. H., and QUINN, J., 'Automobile accidents as an expression of psychopathology in an alcoholic population'. *Quarterly Journal of Studies on Alcohol*, vol. 28, 1967, pp. 505–16.

55. SERVAIS, J. and HUBIN, P., 'Étude psychopharmacologique de l'amphetamine et du meprobamate chez l'homme normal'. *International Journal of Neuropharmacology*, vol. 3, 1964, pp. 517–40.

56. SHAGASS, C., 'Sedation threshold. A neurophysiological tool for psychosomatic research'. *Psychosomatic Medicine*, vol. 18, 1956, pp. 410–19.

57. SHAGASS, C. and JONES, A. L., 'A neurophysiological test for psychiatric diagnosis: results in 750 patients'. *American Journal of Psychiatry*, vol. 114, 1958, pp. 1002–9.

58. SHAGASS, C. and KERENYI, A. B., 'Neurophysiologic studies of

personality'. *Journal of Nervous and Mental Disease*, vol. 126, 1958, pp. 141–7.

59. SHAGASS, C., MIHALIK, J. and JONES, A. L., 'Clinical psychiatric studies using the sedation threshold'. *Journal of Psychosomatic Research*, vol. 2, 1957, pp. 45–55.

60. SHAW, Peter. *The Reflector: Representing Human Affairs, as they are; and may be improved.* Longman, 1750.

61. SLATER, P. E., MORIMOTO, K. and HYDE, R. W., 'The effect of group administration upon symptom formation under LSD'. *Journal of Nervous and Mental Disease*, vol. 125, 1957, pp. 312–21.

62. STARKWEATHER, J. A., 'Individual and situational influences on drug effects'. In FEATHERSTONE, R. M. and SIMON, A. (Eds.), *A Pharmacologic Approach to the Study of the Mind*, 3, C. C. Thomas, Springfield, 1959.

63. STEINBERG, H. and SUMMERFIELD, A., 'Influence of a depressant drug on acquisition in rote learning'. *Quarterly Journal of Experimental Psychology*, vol. 9, 1957, pp. 138–45.

64. STEINBOOK, R. M., JONES, M. B. and AINSLIE, J. D. 'Suggestibility and the placebo response'. *Journal of Nervous and Mental Disease*, vol. 140, 1965, pp. 87–91.

65. STERNBACH, R. A., 'The effects of instructional sets on autonomic responsivity'. *Psychophysiology*, vol. 1, 1964, pp. 67–72.

66. STEVENS, J. M. and DERBYSHIRE, A. J., 'Shifts along the alert-repose continuum during remission of catatonic "stupor" with amobarbital'. *Psychosomatic Medicine*, vol. 20, 1958, pp. 99–107.

67. SUMMERFIELD, A. and STEINBERG, H., 'Reducing interference in forgetting'. *Quarterly Journal of Experimental Psychology*, vol. 9, 1957, pp. 146 –54.

68. TALLAND, G. A. and QUARTON, G. C., 'The effects of drugs and familiarity on performance in continuous visual search'. *Journal of Nervous and Mental Disease*, vol. 143, 1966, pp. 87–91.

69. 'The drugged driver'. *Drive Magazine* (Automobile Association), New Year, 1969.

70. TISSOT, R., 'The effects of certain drugs on the sleep cycle in man'. *Progress in Brain Research*, vol. 18, Elsevier, Amsterdam, 1965.

71. WAYNE, E. J. 'Alcohol and driving – the pharmacological back-

ground'. In *Alcohol and Road Traffic*, British Medical Association, 1963.

72. WHITMAN, R. M., PIERCE, C. M., MAAS, J. W., and BALD-RIDGE, B., 'Drugs and dreams. II. Imipramine and prochlorperazine'. *Comprehensive Psychiatry*, vol. 2, 1961, pp. 219–26.

73. 'Without prescription'. Number 27 in a series of papers on current health problems, Office of Health Economics, 1968.

74. WOLF, S. and WOLFF, H. G. *Human Gastric Function. An Experimental Study of a Man and his Stomach*. Oxford University Press, 1943.

75. *World Health Organization Technical Report Series*, No. 273, 1964.

76. *World Health Organization Technical Report Series*, No. 363, 1967.

77. ZEGANS, L. S., POLLARD, J. C. and BROWN, D., 'The effects of LSD-25 on creativity and tolerance to regression'. *Archives of General Psychiatry*, vol. 16, 1967, pp. 740–9.

Glossary of Drug Names and Types

The following list is intended as a guide to the nomenclature of psychopharmacology. The list is by no means exhaustive but the drugs included are those most commonly encountered, many of which have been referred to in the body of the book. As noted in the Preface, the drug names used in the main entries are those arrived at by the World Health Organization. In this respect special mention should be made of the barbiturates, over which most confusion can arise because of the different names used for the same drug in different countries. The principal difference lies in the name ending preferred, the United States using the ending *-al* (e.g. pentobarbit*al*), whereas in Britain the ending *-one* is used (e.g. pentobarbit*one*). The WHO terminology, and therefore the one used here, follows American usage and equivalent forms will only be given if, as happens with a few barbiturates, the complete name also differs in Britain.

Acetylcholine – Hormonal transmitter in the autonomic and central nervous systems and, as a drug, a parasympathomimetic agent, i.e. a substance that acts by stimulating the parasympathetic division of the autonomic nervous system.

Adrenaline – see *epinephrine*.

Amitriptyline – Antidepressive drug chemically similar to *imipramine*.

Amobarbital – Intermediate-acting barbiturate.

Amphetamines – Group of central nervous stimulants chemically related to *epinephrine*. In the singular *amphetamine* usually refers to *amphetamine sulphate*, the prototype drug of the group.

Amylobarbitone – see *amobarbital*.

Analeptic drugs – Term sometimes used to describe central nervous stimulants.

Ataractic drugs – Term sometimes applied to the tranquillizers, though used inconsistently to cover the major tranquillizers, the minor tranquillizers, or both. Refers to the ability of these drugs to diminish mental disturbance.

Atropine – Parasympatholytic agent, i.e. a drug that acts by blocking the parasympathetic division of the autonomic nervous system.

Barbiturates – Group of sedative/hyponotics derived from barbituric acid. Normally subdivided, according to the length of time they act, into four groups: long-, intermediate-, short-, and ultra-short-acting. Frequently administered as the sodium salt (e.g. *phenobarbital sodium*) for which the shortened name (e.g. *phenobarbital*) is often used.

Bemegride – Drug having a powerful stimulating action on the central nervous system.

Benzodiazepines – Group of minor tranquillizers which includes *chlordiazepoxide* and *diazepam*.

Butyrophenones – Group of compounds with properties similar to those of the *phenothiazines*. The most commonly used example is *haloperidol*.

Cannabis – Active ingredient of the resinous extract (cannabis resin) derived from the flowering female hemp plant.

Chlordiazepoxide – Minor tranquillizer of the *benzodiazepine* group, used in the treatment of anxiety and tension.

Chlorpromazine – First phenothiazine tranquillizer used in the treatment of psychotic illness.

Cyclobarbital – Short-acting barbiturate.

Dexamphetamine – Chemical variant of the prototype *amphetamine* and, compared with the latter, about twice as potent, weight for weight.

Diazepam – Minor tranquillizer of the *benzodiazepine* group, used in the treatment of anxiety and tension.

Epinephrine – Hormone secreted by the adrenal glands and, as a drug, a sympathomimetic agent, i.e. a substance that acts by stimulating the sympathetic division of the autonomic nervous system.

Glutethimide – Sedative/hypnotic chemically related to glutamic acid.

Haloperidol – Major tranquillizer belonging to a group known as *butyrophenones*. Sometimes used particularly in the treatment of mania.

Hashish – One of many synonyms for marihuana or cannabis. Etymologically derived from the Arabic 'hashinan', or herb-eater.

Heroin – Semi-synthetic narcotic derived from *morphine*.

Imipramine – Antidepressive drug markedly different in chemical structure and action from the *monoamineoxidase inhibitors*. Chemically similar to *chlorpromazine*.

Lysergide – lysergic acid diethylamide.

Marihuana – Popular term describing several forms in which *cannabis* is prepared for consumption.

Mepazine – see *pecazine*.

Meprobamate – Minor tranquillizer having muscle relaxant properties and used in the treatment of anxiety and tension.

Methamphetamine – Methyl variant of the prototype *amphetamine*.

Monoamineoxidase inhibitors – Group of antidepressive drugs once thought to have their mood-elevating effect through their action of raising the concentration of brain amines. Well-known for their tendency to cause the 'cheese reaction', a hypertensive side-effect occurring in people eating foodstuffs, such as cheese, which contain high levels of amines.

Morphine – Naturally occurring alkaloid constitutent of opium having powerful narcotic properties.

Neuropletic drugs – Term sometimes used to describe the major tranquillizers.

Noradrenaline – see *norepinephrine*.

Norepinephrine – Hormone secreted at the nerve endings of the sympathetic nervous system, and a neural transmitter in the brain.

Opium – Narcotic derived from the juice of poppy capsules and natural source of the drug *morphine*.

Pecazine – Tranquillizer of the phenothiazine group.

Pentetrazol – Drug having a powerful stimulating action on the central nervous system.

Pentobarbital – Short-acting barbiturate.

Phencyclidine – Drug having psychotomimetic properties.

Phenelzine – An antidepressive drug of the *monoamineoxidase inhibitor* group.

Phenobarbital – Long-acting barbiturate.

Phenothiazines – Group of major tranquillizers of which the most notable example is the prototype drug *chlorpromazine*.

Phentolamine – Sympatholytic agent, i.e. a drug that acts by blocking the sympathetic division of the autonomic nervous system.

Prochloperazine – Tranquillizer of the *phenothiazine* group.

Promazine – Tranquillizer of the *phenothiazine* group. Chemically very similar to, but less potent than, *chlorpromazine*.

Quinalbarbitone – see *secobarbital*.

Rauwolfia alkaloids – Substances derived from Rauwolfia Serpentina, a plant used for centuries in India as a cure for insanity. The plant's principal active constituent is the alkaloid, *reserpine*.

Reserpine – Substance belonging to the group of *Rauwolfia alkaloids*, once, but now little, used as a major tranquillizer in the treatment of schizophrenia.

Secobarbital – Short-acting barbiturate.

Thiopental sodium – Ultra-short-acting barbiturate.

Thymoleptic drugs – Term sometimes used to describe the antidepressive, or 'mood-elevating', drugs.

Trifluoperazine – Tranquillizer of the *phenothiazine* group. Next in importance to *chlorpromazine* as a treatment for psychotic illness.

Index

More about Penguins and Pelicans

Penguinews, which appears every month contains details of all the new books issued by Penguins as they are published. From time to time it is supplemented by *Penguins in Print*, which is a complete list of all available books published by Penguins. (There are well over three thousand of these.)

A specimen copy of *Penguinews* will be sent to you free on request, and you can become a subscriber for the price of the postage. For a year's issues (including the complete lists) please send 30p if you live in the United Kingdom, or 60p if you live elsewhere. Just write to Dept EP, Penguin Books Ltd, Harmondsworth, Middlesex, enclosing a cheque or postal order, and your name will be added to the mailing list.

Note: *Penguinews* and *Penguins in Print* are not available in the U.S.A. or Canada

The Politics of Experience and The Bird of Paradise

R. D. Laing

Is there anywhere such a thing as a *normal* man?

Modern society clamps a straitjacket of conformity on every child who's born. In the process man's potentialities are devastated and the terms 'sanity' and 'madness' become ambiguous. The schizophrenic may simply be someone who has been unable to suppress his normal instincts to conform to an abnormal society.

The whole question of 'normality' is raised in this new book by Dr Laing, the author of *The Divided Self*. In the fog of psychological ambiguities, as he sees it, we cannot rely on the navigators, just because the theories of experts about alienation too often manifest the very faults they describe. The author's argument leads him to explore the psychological weapons of constriction, deprivation, splitting, and projection; and he does not hesitate to call on science, rhetoric, poetry, and polemic to support his points. If he leaves us with little more than the bitter taste of truth in this modern dilemma, at least he believes that 'as long as there are survivors, there is still hope'.

also available

THE DIVIDED SELF
SELF AND OTHERS
and
SANITY, MADNESS AND THE FAMILY
(*with A. Esterson*)

Drugs

Medical, Psychological, and Social Facts

Peter Laurie

SECOND EDITION

What are the known facts about the 'dangerous' drugs?
What actual harm, mental or physical, do they cause?
Which of them are addictive, and how many addicts are
there?

Peter Laurie has talked with doctors, policemen, addicts,
and others intimately involved with this problem. He has
tried some of the drugs for himself and closely studied the
medical literature (including little-known reports of
American research). The result of his inquiries into the
pharmacological uses and social effects of drugs today
appears in this book. Now re-issued in Pelicans, it has
already been through five printings as a Penguin Special.

Originally published before the Wootton report, *Drugs*
was the first objective study to offer all the major medical,
psychological, and social facts about the subject to a
public which is too often fed with alarmist and sensational
reports. For this second edition in Pelicans Peter Laurie
has added fresh information and statistics concerning
English users of drugs and noted changes in the law.

Dreams and Nightmares

J. A. Hadfield

Dreams have a fascination for everyone, partly
because of their bizarre nature, partly because
these strange imaginings come from within
ourselves, and partly because of the effect they
have upon our daily lives. It is not surprising that
efforts at dream interpretation have been made
throughout all ages, by the most primitive tribes,
who regard them as premonitions, no less than in
the attempts at establishing a scientific method
made by Freud with his sexual wish-fulfilment
theory, Jung with his archetypes from the racial
subconscious, and Adler with his urge to power.
In this book, Dr Hadfield attempts to show that
dreams have a biological role, and may be useful
in the solution of the practical everyday, as well as
of the deep-rooted, problems of our life. Many
mathematical problems have been solved in dreams,
and many scientific discoveries made by their
means. We cannot, therefore, afford to ignore the
significance of our dreaming, just as we cannot
afford to ignore that of our intuition. This book,
then, is a brief sketch of the mechanism, nature,
and importance of our dream life.

The Penguin English Library

Thomas De Quincey

Confessions of an English Opium Eater

EDITED BY ALETHEA HAYTER

De Quincey wrote his famous *Confessions* at a time when opium was as easily available as aspirin today, and almost as frequently used, and when its dangers were not understood. Though something of a fugitive from respectable society, he shared his addiction with some of the most distinguished men of his age. But the *Confessions* are not about drug-addiction. 'They are a meditation on the mechanism of the imagination, an exploration of the interior life of an altogether exceptional being.' Brilliantly gifted and charming, De Quincey suffered from what he himself called a 'chronic passion of anxiety' which led him from the security and success he might have enjoyed into the direst poverty, and into the experiences which form the subjects of the terrible, drug-induced dreams he describes so superbly.